THE
WEEKEND ATHLETE'S
FITNESS GUIDE

THE WEEKEND ATHLETE'S FITNESS GUIDE

by
Peter Verney

Facts On File
119 W. 57th Street, New York, N.Y. 10019

THE WEEKEND ATHLETE'S FITNESS GUIDE

First published in the United States in 1980 by Facts On File, Inc.

Library of Congress Cataloging in Publication Data

Verney, Peter, 1930-
  Sports fitness.

  Bibliography: p. 251
  1. Sports—Safety measures. 2. Physical fitness.
3. Sports—Training. I. Title.
GV344.V47   616.02′52   79-25346
ISBN 0-87196-301-9

10 9 8 7 6 5 4 3 2 1
Printed in the United States of America

197637

Contents

For a more specific breakdown, see the page guides that introduce each section.

Acknowledgments

Very many people and sports institutions on both sides of the Atlantic have assisted me during the writing of this book, and I would like to take this opportunity of expressing my gratitude for all their help. I would especially like to thank those who gave me advice over the medical aspects of sports fitness: Dr. Ken Chekofsky of the Institute of Sports Medicine, New York; Dr. Alan Maryon-Davis, medical officer of the Health Education Council, London, and Drs. Hubert and Bessy Crouch of Eastcombe, Gloucestershire.

My thanks are also due to my designers Patricia Pillay and Pete Pengilley; illustrators Maggie Raynor and Clive Spong, who have done a magnificent job; and to my editor Diane Flanel, for her skill, knowledge and inspiration.

None of this, however, would have been possible without the wholehearted and unselfish cooperation of the many coaches, trainers and players who helped me in the course of my research. I would particularly like to thank:

Elizabeth Adams (riding); Gordon Adams (long jump); Dr. Ian Adams (marathon); John Adams (archery); Paul Adlington (water skiing); Richard Aronson (gymnastics); Ron Balls (lacrosse); Philip Barthott (hurdling); Dr. J. Betts (snorkel and scuba); John Blewitt (speed skating); Art Bloomfield (baseball); Tim Bonsor (sprinting); Brian Brain (cricket); Andy Brassington (cricket); Mike Briers (team handball); Mike Cannon (diving); Geoff Capes (shot put); Mike Carley (boxing); Frank Charnock (fencing); David Clements (figure skating); Michael Close (table tennis); Brian Coleman (basketball); Frank Costello (hurdling); Ian Cundy (lacrosse); O. A. Cussen (badminton); Dave Dash (skateboarding); George Dimmer (surfing); John Else (cycling); Ron Emes (canoeing); Paul Fernandez (baseball); Mrs. M. P. French (netball); Paddy Garratt (swimming); Julian Goater (middle distance); Vonnie Gros (field hockey); Jeffrey Gutteridge (pole vault); John Hantz (lacrosse); Christopher Harrison (javelin); R. B. Hawkey (squash); Alex Hay (golf); D. J. Hayward (triple jump); Derek Healy (speed skating); David Heller (swimming); Peter Hicks (roller skating); W. Holland (weight lifting); Ron Holman (long distance); H. I. Jacobs (wrestling); Barry James (windsurfing); R. H. Johnson (squash); Lionel Jones (tennis); Peter Jones (surfing); Steve and Lisa Jordan (badminton); Leo E. Keenan Jr. (golf); Dr. R. W. Kind (archery); Darwin Kingsley (squash); John Lakeman (basketball); Ron Ludington (figure skating); Dr. C. Mack (karate); Peter Marlow (road walking); W. Marlow (sprinting); John Miller (cricket and soccer); Paul Millman (squash); John Moore (skiing); Ted A. Nash (rowing); Dr. F. S. Nelson (figure skating); Chester Nobbs (racquetball); Dr. Noel O'Brien (rowing); Mrs. Ann Palmer (lacrosse); David Partridge (cricket); R. W. E. Poole (cycling); Mike Procter (cricket); Tony Reay (judo); Bev Risman (tennis); John Rost (ice hockey); Rip Rowley (softball); Terry Sancher (racquetball); D. Shelley (marathon); Don Smallwood (baseball); Phil Spicer (water polo); Don Stamp (archery); Annette Stapleton (gymnastics); Ian Stevenson (windsurfing); Barry Swann (volleyball); Raymond Taylor (aikido); Martin Thomas (water polo); Rob Van Mesdag (rowing); David Vinson (field hockey); Richard Wait (rowing); John Waite (judo); Frank Westrell (cycling); Norman Willis (netball); Mike Winch (discus); J. D. Wood (water skiing); Stan Woollam (sailing); Yoshisada Yonezuka (judo).

Introduction

Exercise is bunk. If you are healthy, you don't need it. If you are sick, you shouldn't take it!

HENRY FORD

MANY PEOPLE UNDOUBTEDLY feel the same way as Henry Ford, yet authorities in the medical, educational and social fields believe that exercise is essential, particularly for those who live sedentary lives. This is a message which has been taken up by millions of people around the world who jog, run, walk, do calisthenics or go to fitness classes—all for the sake of exercise.

Many of us, however, find these pursuits boring and monotonous and, if we engage in any exercise at all, we do so by playing sports of all kinds. But whether we concentrate on a single sport or take part in several different ones, all of us would like to improve our performance and increase the enjoyment we get from sport. We can do this by attaining sports fitness—the capacity to play to the limit of one's skill, without fatigue and with a reduced rate of injury.

In the United States, fitness has been defined by the President's Council on Physical Fitness as "the ability to carry out daily tasks efficiently with enough energy left to enjoy leisure-time pursuits and to meet unforeseen emergencies." The definition points to the fact that there is a close relationship between physical fitness and mental alertness. Fitness lowers nervous tension and helps one tolerate physical and emotional stress. The fit have stronger hearts and regular exercise reduces the risk of heart disease. Fitness alone won't give you health, but it will make you less susceptible to sickness. A fit body is also an efficient body, and a fit person will take less time to recover from illness. He or she will also be able to stave off fatigue longer and

7

use less energy for any given job. Above all, a fit person is more likely to sleep well, look well and feel well.

Sports fitness alone won't make you an Olympic champion, but it will give you an edge over your opponents. In sport, confidence is all-important, and basic all-around fitness helps to nurture the confidence that fatigue, muscle pulls and strains are less likely and that you can exert extra effort without pain.

How is sports fitness obtained? Not by constant undirected exercise prolonged until exhaustion sets in, but by a carefully regulated routine—a routine that is balanced between over- and undertraining and that carefully combines periods of exercise with periods of rest, to "recharge the batteries" and revitalize the body.

Fitness involves the fine tuning of a highly complex machine—the human body—and it means training, both for general conditioning and, more specifically, for one's chosen sport. Most of us, however, have neither the time nor the opportunity to go to a gymnasium or to work with a coach; for us, sport or exercise means an occasional evening, more probably only a weekend workout. If this description fits *you*—that is, if you see yourself as a part-time or weekend sportsperson, and would like to improve your performance at the same time as you safeguard yourself against injury—then this book should put you well on your way.

HOW THIS BOOK WORKS

The Weekend Athlete's Fitness Guide is divided into three parts. **Part I, General Conditioning,** is devoted to showing the casual athlete how to attain a general standard of all-around fitness and conditioning, a foundation on which specific sports fitness may later be built.

Here at the outset you must determine—via a series of simple fitness tests provided on p. 12—whether or not you are fit enough to take part in unaccustomed exercise, either for the first time or after a prolonged lay-off. This is particularly important for anyone over 30 or anyone with certain medical conditions; consultation with a doctor may be crucial in some cases, as will be explained in this part.

For most people, these simple fitness tests will be a mere formality, and from the outset you will, no doubt, be ready to take part in most, if not all, sports. The next step is to show you how to attain a reasonable standard in the three main areas of all-round fitness: flexibility in the joints and muscles; a degree of general body strength; and a fair level of heart and lung endurance (or stamina). A wide range of exercises is included for each of these categories, from which you can take your pick, depending on your own individual exercise preferences and specific fitness needs. To help you knit together these exercises into a balanced fitness regime, some sample home exercise circuits are included as well as an explanation of popular training routines practiced by top teams and individual coaches and athletes. Rounding off Part I is advice on the all-important warm-up and a few tips on diet and pre-exercise eating.

Part II, Sport by Sport, outlines the physical demands of each sport, as well as providing suggestions for alternative or off-season sports that players may find beneficial to their chosen game. Specific conditioning and warm-up routines are included to show you how to build up specific fitness for each sport, and finally each sport ends with a discussion of the injuries and conditions associated with it.

Part III, Sports Injuries, expands on the injury information in Part II. The first two sections here cover simple ailments, conditions and injuries which can be dealt with by home treatment, and a final section deals with on-the-spot first aid for emergencies that might arise.

PART I
General Conditioning

Fit for Sport?

SOME AUTHORITIES SUGGEST that a medical examination should be obligatory before imposing strenuous or unaccustomed exercise on the human body. Others say that anyone over 30 should have a checkup. Others propose a stress electrocardiogram. The British Royal College of Physicians and the British Cardiac Society counsel, however, that:

> Most people do not need a medical examination before starting an exercise program. There are no risks in regular dynamic exercise as long as the program begins gently and only gradually increases in vigor. Older persons, the obese, and those with a history of cardiovascular disease or symptoms, should first consult their doctor. Those who develop unexpected symptoms during exercise should also seek medical advice.

More specifically, most authorities are agreed that if you are suffering from or have ever suffered from any of the following conditions, you should have a thorough medical exam:

- high blood pressure or heart disease;
- chest troubles, such as asthma or bronchitis;
- arthritis or pains in the joints or back.

In addition, you will need to consult your doctor if you are still recovering from an operation or long illness, or—and this is most important of all—if you have any other health worries that you feel might be worsened by exercise.

If at any time during exercise you feel distress such as nausea, headache, breathlessness, pounding in the head, dizziness, trembling or pain in the chest, *stop immediately*. This is a clear indication that you have gone beyond the limits of your present physical exercise tolerance. These distress signals should wear off very shortly; if they do not you should see a doctor without delay.

FITNESS TESTING

An exercise program should start gradually. The following is a simple series of stamina tests designed to show whether or not you are fit enough to start taking part regularly in the sport or sports of your choice. (Whatever your current level of fitness, a sensible and gradual increase in playing intensity is always advisable—especially at the start of a season or after a prolonged lay-off.)

Test 1. Step Walking

Walk up and down a flight of stairs (15–20 steps is ideal). Do this 3 times fairly briskly. If you are not panting or puffing, proceed to Test 2.

If you are out of breath or have difficulty holding a normal conversation after this exercise, then you should consult a doctor about starting an exercise and/or walking program under medical supervision.

Test 2. Jogging in Place

Your feet should rise at least 6 inches from the floor. Keep jogging until you begin to feel a bit out of breath or your leg muscles begin to ache, then stop. Don't overdo it. You should manage 3 minutes comfortably (if over 50, then 2 minutes). If you can do this, proceed to Test 3.

If you cannot, consult a doctor or start a gentle walking fitness program to gradually build up your stamina. (This should entail walking over gradually increasing distances. At first walk slowly for a short distance. Then, as you become fitter, walk further and more briskly.)

Test 3. Step-Ups

Using a strong chair (or the second step of a flight of stairs), step up and down briskly, using alternate feet. Stop as soon as you feel out of breath or your muscles begin to ache. Again, don't overdo it. You should manage 3 minutes and still be able to carry on a conversation (over-50, 2 minutes). If you can, proceed to the final test.

If you cannot, set about your own walking fitness program.

Test 4. Jogging

Jog gently, without any hurry, for 1 mile. Your times should read:

Men under 45—10 minutes
Men over 45—add 2 minutes for every 5 years
(Women should add 2 minutes to these times.)

Note: During the test and afterwards you should be able to hold a normal conversation. If you cannot, you should start a walking program (*see* Test 2 *above*) and then progress to an alternate walking and jogging routine 2-3 times a week: start with 100 yards walking, then 100 yards jogging, then walk again and so on. As you get fitter pare down the walking and increase the jogging until you can comfortably jog the necessary distance without distress.

When you can do this, you are ready for sport—or rather *most* sports, as some are particularly strenuous and should be eased into gradually (e.g., squash or football).

PULSE RATE

An alternative fitness test is to use your pulse rate as an indicator—at first while at rest, and then after specific and calculated exercise.

To take the pulse, turn your left hand palm upwards and place two fingers of the right hand on the left wrist about 3 inches below the mound of the palm. You should then be able to feel your pulse as the blood passes through the artery. Look at your watch and for a period of 15 seconds count the number of pulses. Multiply by 4 to give your pulse rate per minute.

Take your first reading after sitting quietly for a few minutes.

Then stand in front of a pile of large books 8 inches high (a bench, box or step of similar height will do). Place your left foot on the books, then step on to it with both feet. Step down again, first with your left foot and then with the right. Repeat for 3 minutes at a rate of 24 steps per minute (look at your watch while doing this). Wait for 1 minute after the exercise, then test your pulse again. Check your rating with the table below. (Bear in mind that the lower the pulse rate, the fitter you generally are.)

Note: If you feel any distress while doing this test, *stop immediately.*

	MEN	*WOMEN*
Excellent	*Up to 68*	*Up to 76*
Good	*68–79*	*76–85*
Average	*80–89*	*86–94*
Below Average	*90–99*	*95–109*
Very Poor	*More than 100*	*More than 110*

If your score is Average or better, it should be quite all right for you to take up exercise right away. If you score Below Average or Very Poor, consult your doctor before taking on any new exercise.

SPECIAL CASES

Men and Women over 50

Without exercise, the body declines more rapidly with age. Blood pressure rises as fatty deposits clog the arteries. Lung capacity decreases and the chest wall loses flexibility, reducing the amount of oxygen available to the body tissue. The muscles gradually lose strength, and activity involving muscular endurance becomes more difficult. The percentage of body fat rises; the body's capacity to do work declines with increasing rapidity; and reflexes and speed of movement slow down.

Regular exercise won't halt the aging process altogether, but it may help to delay many of its effects. Among other things exercise will:

- strengthen the heart and lungs;
- enhance vigor and vitality;
- reduce fatigue; and
- give a general sense of over-all well-being.

Most of the exercises that appear later in this chapter can be performed safely—and with great physical benefit—by people over 50. Similarly, there are many sports that are suitable for this age group, but there are others in which it is unwise for the over-50s to take part unless they have been doing them on a fairly regular basis for much of their lives.

Thus, if you are over 50, before taking up any form of strenuous exercise or new sport (and that includes one that you haven't played for many years), it is obligatory that you consult your doctor.

If you are given the go-ahead, be sure to break yourself in to the new (or resumed) exercise with care and common sense.

Women in Sport

Most of the ancient myths about women in sport have long since passed away, and there are very few sports which are still the exclusive reserve of the male. Physiologically this is quite understandable, for in physical fitness terms women are not all that different from men.

In general, women are lighter than men and have less lean body weight and some 10 per cent more fat then their male counterparts. Men do possess nearly twice as much muscle bulk as women and therefore more pure strength; however, when muscle size is compared with body size, strength is basically the same for women as for men. Women have the edge over men with regard to general suppleness; however, they tend to be more susceptible to injury, particularly "soft-tissue" injuries such as bruising, sprains and strains.

Pregnancy: Playing sports while pregnant is now accepted as not only practicable, but positively beneficial—provided that caution is observed, particularly during the first 3 months and last 2 months of term. Sport in most cases tones and strengthens the lower back and abdominal muscles, and as such is particularly desirable in pregnancy. However, *no sustained exercise* *or sport should be undertaken without prior consultation with a doctor.*

There are some sports, it should be noted, that are generally held to be more undesirable than others to continue during pregnancy. In general, these include any that involve considerable pelvic or back movement, and those that common sense dictates are obviously unwise to take part in to the same degree of strenuousness to which you have been accustomed.

Among specific sports to be avoided are:

- Golf, especially in the last 3 months, due to risk of back injury resulting from ligaments loosened prior to delivery;
- Field-throwing events in athletics, due to the twisting action and hip rotation employed;
- Gymnastics, which is simply too rigorous;
- Fencing, which can result in overstretching;
- Skiing (both water and snow), which could result in complications after falls; and
- Riding, because of the danger of falls and too vigorous shaking.

Swimming, on the other hand, is particularly safe, as well as beneficial, as the water bears up the body weight.

It is generally unwise to take up new sports during pregnancy, especially those that make considerable demands on stamina or those that involve a lot of stretching. In case of spotting or pains before time—or anything else out of the ordinary occurring (even if it is only a feeling of unease)—*stop immediately* and consult your doctor.

A Balanced Fitness

A FAIR STANDARD of general fitness is the first essential for anyone taking part in sport. Sports skills are founded on specific fitness for a given sport, but without a basic level of general fitness in the first place there is no foundation on which to build. Although fitness for tennis is quite different to the fitness required for weight lifting, both sports demand a basic level of all-around fitness. Without it an athlete is unable to utilize a specific skill to the full extent; he or she will tire more easily and in turn will be more prone to injury. The aim of this section, therefore, is to point the way to achieving and developing a balanced fitness for the whole body.

Attaining sports fitness is largely a matter of individual preference; thus a wide choice of possible exercises are listed below. From these you may make a selection and construct a program to suit your needs. It cannot be emphasized too strongly, however, that these are only the building blocks from which to construct the "house" of your choice. What "style" of house is needed for those taking part in specific sports we will examine in Part II, "Sport by Sport."

There are 3 exercise components that go into planning a program for attaining a balanced fitness: **flexibility, or mobility, exercises**, designed to loosen stiff joints and muscles, and ensure that they can be moved through their full range; **strength exercises**, to develop muscular strength and muscle endurance; and **heart and lung exercises**—sometimes called **cardiovascular (CV) or cardiorespiratory (CR) exercises**—to build stamina and endurance.

Note: Your workouts should be on a regular, sustained basis, involving more than just a few token exercises. Make your exercise sessions purposeful and progressive. Exercise can be fun, but use discretion. On the other hand, don't be afraid to break into a sweat.

The **repetitions and/or durations** suggested for each exercise are the lowest at which it is felt that the exercise can be of actual benefit. Most reasonably fit people will find that they can increase the suggested repetitions or durations without distress, *but this should be done gradually*.

The **exercise code letters** in the following sections will be repeated throughout the book.

FLEXIBILITY EXERCISES

The flexibility exercises below are designed to loosen and limber up the joints and make the body more supple. Some of these exercises feature in the general warm-up program (*see* p. 40–41), the need for which is now accepted by athletes and coaches alike as an essential procedure before a training workout or game. Others feature in yoga routines or similar regimens that promote relaxation for the body and mind.

Ideally these exercises should be practiced 3–4 times a day if you have the time. But take it easy, especially if you are unfit. Joint flexibility should be attained gradually. Bear in mind that some people's joints are more naturally flexible than others, and that there is a loss of flexibility during aging.

When doing these exercises, stretch gently and gradually—but not to the point of pain—until a position of maximum flex is reached. *Do not bob or bounce*. Hold the position for 5–10 seconds, then relax and repeat.

HIPS AND THIGHS	TRUNK AND NECK
F1. Side Bends (Lateral Bending)	**F2. Trunk Twists**

HIPS AND THIGHS

F1. Side Bends (Lateral Bending)

Stand erect, feet comfortably apart, hands at sides. Bend trunk to left and slide hand down the thigh as far as is comfortable. Return to upright position. Repeat on other side.

Note: Keep the back straight.

Repetitions: 6 each side, increasing to 10

TRUNK AND NECK

F2. Trunk Twists

Stand erect, feet comfortably apart, hands on hips. Twist alternately from side to side.

Note: Keep the back straight. At each twist try to look as far over the shoulder as possible.

Repetitions: 6 each side, increasing to 10

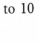
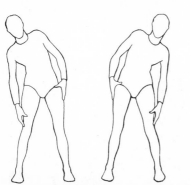
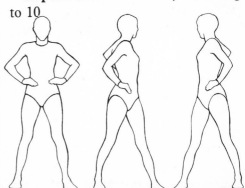

BACK, SHOULDERS AND ARMS
F3. Alternate Toe Touches

Stand erect, feet comfortably apart, arms raised. Reach down and touch right hand to left toe, return to the fully upright position with back straight, then touch left hand to right toe.

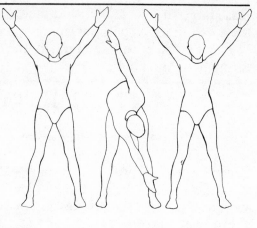

Note: Keep legs as straight as possible and do not rotate the hips. Return to the fully upright position with the back straight after each movement. If you cannot reach all the way down to the toes, reach as far down the leg as is comfortable. After a while the back will become more supple and you will find that you can reach further and further toward the opposite feet.

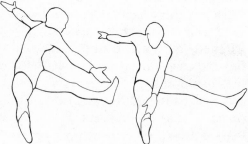

An alternative is to carry out the exercise sitting down.

Repetitions: 5 each side, increasing to 10

NECK
F.4 Neck Rolls

Stand erect, feet comfortably apart, hands on hips. Drop chin to your chest and then roll the head round, pushing the head back and raising the chin. Repeat in a continuous movement clockwise, then counterclockwise.

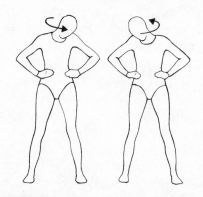

Note: Stand erect throughout and keep the stomach in.

Repetitions: 5

SHOULDERS
F5. Shoulder Shrugs

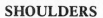

Stand erect, feet comfortably apart, arms hanging loosely at the sides. Raise shoulders up to the ears, then relax and push them as far down as possible.

Repetitions: 10, rising to 20

F6. Wing Stretchers

Stand erect, feet comfortably apart, elbows at shoulder level with fists clenched in front of the body. Force the elbows back as far as they will go, count to 2 then relax.

Note: The body must remain upright throughout. Do not arch the back. Keep the head erect.

Repetitions: 10, rising to 20

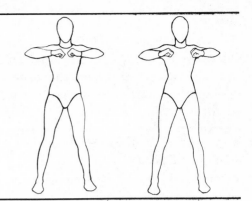

ARMS AND UPPER BODY

F7. Arm Circles

Stand erect, feet comfortably apart, arms held forward at shoulder height. Bring the arms upward brushing past the ears, then around and return to the starting position.

A variation of this exercise is to hold the arms out sideways, level with the shoulders, and describe small circling movements, gradually getting larger until the arms brush past the ears in full swing.

Note: Practice both forward and backward. Flex and rotate the wrist and flex the fingers during the exercise.

Repetitions: 10, rising to 20

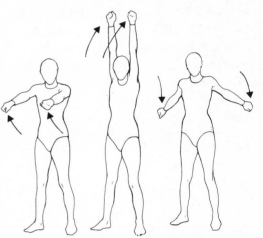

F8. Arm Flings

Stand erect, feet comfortably apart, arms held at shoulder height with elbows bent so the fingers just touch. Fling left arm outward, then return to the center; then the right arm, returning to the center. Repeat.

Note: Body and head must remain erect throughout. Hold in stomach, and do not rotate the hips. Force the arm back at each fling.

Repetitions: 10

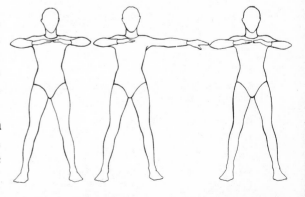

WRISTS
F9. Wrist Shakes
Standing or sitting, hold arms out, let the hands drop, then shake the wrists and hands upwards, downwards and sideways.

Note: Try to keep the forearm still.
Duration: 15–20 seconds

STOMACH, THIGH AND CALF
F10. The Reach
Stand erect, feet comfortably apart, hands loosely at the sides. Breathe in deeply and slowly bend backward, thrusting out the pelvis. At the same time reach upward with the hands, fingers outstretched. Breathe out. Hold position for 5 seconds before returning to the upright position. Breathe in deeply and repeat.
Repetitions: 10

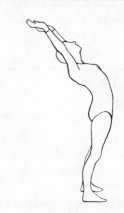

GROIN AND THIGH
(including Quadriceps and Hamstrings)

Note: F12 is excellent for stretching the hamstrings; **F14** is particularly good for the quadriceps. **F11** and **F13** exercise both sets of thigh muscles.

F11. The Lunge (Sideways Splits/Fencing)
This is an excellent exercise for increasing stride length. Stand erect, feet comfortably apart, hands on hips. Pivot feet outward and then take a stride with the right foot and adopt a lunging position as in fencing (*see* illustration). Keep pushing the left leg back and keep it straight, while at the same time pressing the body toward the floor. Hold for a count of 5 seconds, relax. Repeat on the other side.

Note: The back should remain straight throughout and the forward leg vertical.

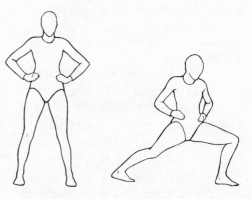

Repetitions: 5 each side, increasing to 10

F12. Hurdles (Sitting Stretch)

Sit on floor as shown, with right leg outstretched and left leg at a right angle, bent back (*see* illustration). Place hands at top of right leg and slide them down toward the foot, bending the body, neck and head as close to the knee as possible. Relax. Repeat a number of times, then change legs.

Note: At first you may not be able to reach very far down the extended leg, but this will improve with practice. Do not overstretch, and do not bounce. Apply a steady pressure and then relax. Try to keep the extended leg close to the floor.

Repetitions: 5 each leg, increasing to 10

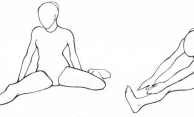

UPPER LEG
F13. Leg Swings

Stand erect, feet together, arms outstretched. For balance hold on to a chair or table at about waist height. Swing the outside leg backward and forward. Relax, repeat on other side.

Note: The body should remain upright.

Repetitions: 10, increasing to 20 each side

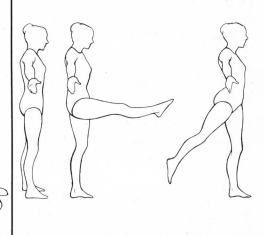

LOWER LEG

F14. Knee Pulls (Knee Hug/Knee Lift)

Lying flat on the ground, pull each knee alternately (a), or both knees together (b), in to the chest. Hold for count of 5, then return leg to floor. The head may either remain on the floor or be hunched forward (as shown).

Alternatively, stand erect and lift the right knee as high as you can and clasp it to the chest. Hold for a count of 5, and return foot to ground. Relax. Repeat with other leg.

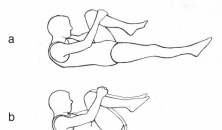

Note: The body should remain upright, the back straight.

Repetitions: 5 each leg, increasing to 10

F15. Calf Stretches

Stand at arm's length away from a wall with feet together and hands touching. Then lean forward, bending the arms and keeping the feet *flat* on the floor. Straighten, relax.

Note: The purpose of this exercise is to stretch the calf muscles, so it is essential to keep the feet flat on the floor and the back straight. You can also use this exercise to strengthen the fingers by pushing the body upright again with fingers alone.

Repetitions: 5, increasing to 10

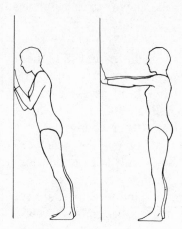

General Flexibility Exercise Routines

In addition to flexibility exercises, a variety of routines are also practiced by athletes. A few of these are listed below. Many are also excellent aids to heart and lung fitness. It is important to carry out a warming-up program (*see* pp. 40–41) before starting these routines to avoid strains and sprains.

The Shuttle Run

This is an activity designed to develop the start-stop and quick-change-of-direction agility needed in many sports such as basketball, football, rugby, hockey and racquet games. In particular it is useful for promoting the quick kick-off, the ability to turn and the rhythm of striding.

There are many versions of the shuttle run, but most are geared to the distances covered during a movement of play in a game. For instance, cross-court moves in tennis rarely cover much more than 10 feet (but you may have to cover up to 40 feet); in baseball the optimum distance is about 20 yards; in rugby 10–15 yards.

Shuttle runs can be laid out either indoors or outdoors. The first requirement is to lay out a baseline and from there pace out a series of distances to be covered. The athlete then starts at the baseline and runs to a mark, turns and runs back. This can be done in the form of a competition with other players or against the clock.

Zigzags

These are intended to develop the side-to-side agility needed in some sports. They involve dashing from side to side over a comparatively short distance.

In laying out a zigzag the only requirement is to have two parallel straight lines the necessary distance apart. A wall is sometimes used to give extra kick-off on one side, but the jarring effect is considerable and you may do yourself damage if the exercise is carried out at too high speed.

Flexibility Sports

In addition to the above exercises, the following sports are excellent for improving all-around flexibility of the body:

Swimming ● Fencing ● Gymnastics ● Squash ● Racquetball ● Volleyball
Judo ● Aikido

STRENGTH EXERCISES

The following exercises are designed primarily to strengthen muscles and ligaments. Muscle power involves two qualities: muscle force, such as that needed by the wrestler, weight lifter and shot putter; and muscle endurance, as required by the swimmer, long-distance runner and football, rugby or soccer player.

Strengthening exercises work on the "overload" principle of gradually increasing repetitions or resistance, or both, to build up the power and often the size of the muscles.

A great variety of exercise permutations are possible, and you should work out a routine which suits your own needs. However, two rules are invariable:

1. Training should be progressive, the work load being gradually increased.
2. To prevent pulled muscles, adequate warm-up exercises (*see* pp. 40ff) should be carried out before exercising.

If possible, carry out your routine daily.

BODY
S1. Push-Ups (Dips)

Lie on the floor face down, legs together, hands under the shoulders. Push body off the floor by straightening the arms. Lower body to the floor by bending the arms. Other variations using a stool are possible (*see* illustrations).

Note: On bending the arms, the body should not quite touch the floor. Keep the back, hips and legs straight.

Repetitions: Start where you comfortably can and increase gradually. (If too difficult, start with modified push-ups.)

The Modified (Knee) Push-Up is advisable for women and children or for the unfit at the start of an exercise routine. It is similar to the push-up except that the body pushes upwards from the knees rather than the toes. It is easier (and less exhausting) because it places less strain on the back and abdomen.

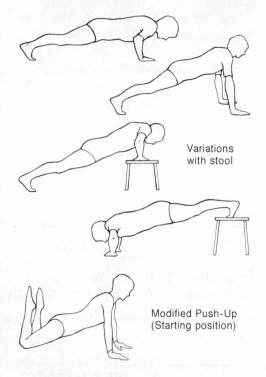

Variations with stool

Modified Push-Up (Starting position)

Repetitions: Start with 5; increase steadily.

ARMS AND SHOULDERS
S2. Pull-Ups (Chins, Chin-Ups)

Find a strong bar just out of reach of the raised arms. Jump up and grasp it—either with palms facing you or facing away (as shown). Hang for a moment, then slowly pull the body upward until the chin is level with the hands. Slowly relax and repeat.

Note: Keep the legs and feet together and try not to sway. At first (particularly if you are overweight), you may find it difficult to do even 1 pull-up, but perseverance and the gradual strengthening of shoulders, arms and hands will make it possible.

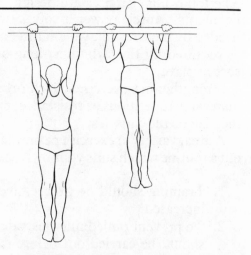

Repetitions: Start where you comfortably can and increase gradually.

S3. Two-Chair Push-Ups

Take 2 kitchen-type chairs with strong legs. Place them as shown, and rest a hand on each. At first accustom the arms to taking the weight of the body by raising the legs off the floor. Then rest and relax. Repeat. When the arms get stronger, start bending and straightening them until a full push-up can be achieved.

Note: Try to keep the body upright; the tendency is to bend forward. Keep the legs well clear of the ground.

Repetitions: Start where you comfortably can and increase gradually

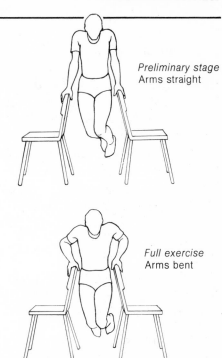

*Preliminary stage
Arms straight*

*Full exercise
Arms bent*

S4. Hip Raises

Sit on the ground, legs and feet together. Place hands to the side, palms flat on the ground; then raise the body, using only the hands, until the arms are straight. Hold for a count of 5, then lower and relax. When this becomes too easy, place hands on a pile of books (which you can add to as you become more proficient), and repeat as before.

Note: Keep the body vertical. Arms should be completely straight and you should not sway. This is also an excellent office exercise and can be done when seated on a chair.

Repetitions: 5, increasing to 10

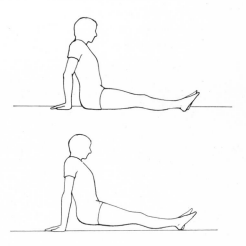

WRIST AND ARMS
S5. Broomstick Roll

Take a length of broomstick, or other stick or rod around 1 inch in diameter and 2 feet long. Tie a length of string to the center just long enough so that it dangles 3–4 inches short of the floor when the stick is at shoulder height. Tie a weight to the loose end—a bundle of books, brick, stone, can of paint, etc., will do the trick. Then, using both hands, palms down, wind the string around the stick. At first carry out the exercise with elbows bent and arms close in to the chest. When you can do this easily, try the exercise with your arms extended straight out in front of you. When the weight reaches the top, *slowly* wind it down until the string is at full extension again.

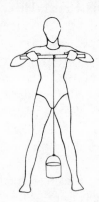

Note: Hold the body erect with back straight during the exercise. The string may slip around the stick, in which case either bore a hole through the center of the stick and thread the string through it, or place a tack through the string to stop it slipping.

Repetition: 6 rolls, increasing to 10

S6. Tennis Ball Squeeze

Take a tennis ball or rubber ball in the hand and squeeze it as hard as you can. Hold the squeeze for a count of 5, then relax and repeat.

Note: Squeeze as hard as you can until you feel your stomach muscles contract. A variation of this exercise is to hold the tennis ball in front of the body, with the elbows parallel to the ground and the fingers of both hands interlocking. Then squeeze the ball as hard as you can until you feel the effect in the shoulder muscles. Hold for a count of 5, relax and then repeat.

Repetitions: 5 squeezes, increasing to 10

FINGERS
S7. Fingertip Push-Ups (Modified Fingertip Push-Ups)

This is an adaptation of the Push-Up or Modified Push-Up (S1). Instead of using the flat of the hands to push up the body, use the fingertips instead.

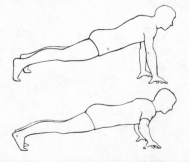

S8. Fingertip Hip Raises
This is an adaptation of the Hip Raise (S4), using the fingers rather than the flat of the hand.

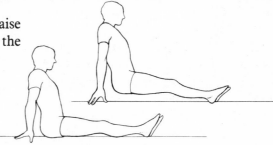

ABDOMEN
S9. "Bicycling"
Lie on the back as shown and perform a "bicycling" motion with the legs.

Note: Carry out the bicycling slowly; thoroughly pull the knee back toward the face and then fully straighten the leg.

Duration: This is a very exhausting exercise for the unfit. Start at 10 seconds and increase in units of 5

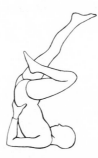

S10. Bent-Leg Sit-Ups
Lie on the back, legs bent, arms to the side. Place feet, about 1 foot apart, under a low sofa, chair or other piece of furniture (or get someone to hold your ankles). Then *slowly* raise the body to a sitting position and lean forward, trying to touch the head to the knees. *Slowly* return to the lying position.

A variation of this exercise is to carry out the sit-up and at the top to do a trunk twist to either side. A more strenuous alternative is to hold the position halfway up.

Note: Do not use the hands to lever yourself upward; some people place them behind the neck to remove temptation. At first you may not get off the floor at all, but with gentle perseverance you will succeed. Later carry out

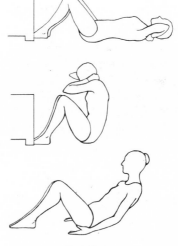

Variation

the exercise without putting the feet under a chair.

Repetitions: Increase in units of 1

27

THIGHS
S11. Half Squats

Stand erect, feet comfortably apart, hands on hips. Rise on the toes and *slowly* sink down, bending the knees until the half-squat position is reached. Hold for a count of 5. Rise again and return to the starting position. Repeat.

Note: Keep the body upright at all times; the tendency is to lean forward. Do *not* go lower than the half-squat position—the full squat places undue strain on the back.

Repetitions: 5, increasing to 10

Note: S11 and S14 are excellent exercises for strengthening the quadriceps. S17 is excellent for the hamstrings.

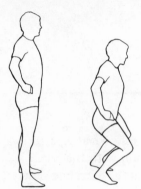

S12. Squat Thrusts (Burpees, Double-Legged Treadmill)

Start as shown, shoot the legs back into the Push-Up position, and then forward again. Repeat.

Note: Keep the feet together and extend them fully on the backward movement.

Repetitions: This is an exercise usually carried out at high speed. Start slowly at the rate of 6 per 15 seconds, then increase rate and duration.

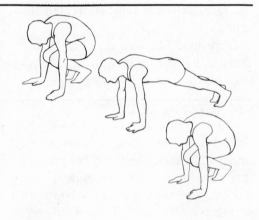

S13. Sprinters (Starts)

This is an excellent exercise to improve stride length and speed on to the ball. It is a variation of the Squat Thrust (S12), but using only one leg at a time.

Note: Change legs rapidly, keeping back straight.

Repetitions: Start slowly with 3 double-leg movements per 15 seconds

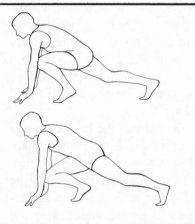

S14. Paint Can Raises

Sitting on a chair or bench, with the thighs parallel to the ground and the lower legs at right angles, take a paint can (or object of similar weight) and hook it on to the toe of one foot. *Slowly* raise the weight until the leg is straight, then *slowly* return it to the ground. Repeat a few times, then change the weight to the other foot.

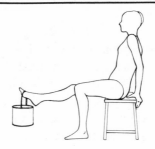

Note: Keep the knees together. To start with, it may help to hold on to the chair or bench; this will become unnecessary later.

Repetitions: 5, increasing to 10

S15. Leg Raises

Lie flat on the back, hands on the floor, palms down. Slowly raise one leg off the ground about 9 inches. Let it return to the floor again and relax. Repeat with the other leg. As you become more proficient, raise the legs higher.

Double Leg Raises: When you feel you are ready, carry out the exercise with both legs.

A further variation is the **Side Leg Raise.**

Note: Keep absolutely flat on the floor. Do not raise the head. Using the hands to help lever the legs upward will help at first, but later should be resisted.

Repetitions: 5, increasing to 10. At that point try the Double-Leg Raise

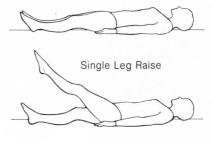

Single Leg Raise

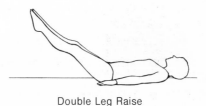

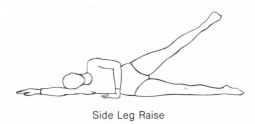

Double Leg Raise

Side Leg Raise

S16. Step-Ups

Stand erect, hands at sides, facing a stool. (A pile of books, bench or other object 12–18 inches high can be substituted.) Place the right foot on the stool and, using only the power of the right leg, raise the body until you are standing with both legs on the seat. Step down again slowly. Change to the left leg and repeat.

Note: Keep the body upright; there is a tendency to lurch forward. At first put the whole foot on the chair seat. Later use only the front part of the foot.

Repetitions: 3, increasing to 10

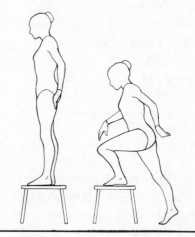

S17. Bench Jumps

Stand alongside a bench, or a pile of books or bricks about 9 inches high and then, with feet together, jump sideways over the obstacle and then back again. You can increase the height as you become more proficient. With proficiency and fitness the style of jump can vary as much as with rope exercises (*see* pp. 33–34). Carried out at speed, bench jumps are also a very good heart and lung exercise.

LOWER LEG
S18. Shin Strengtheners

This is an adaptation of the Paint Can Raise (S14). Sit on the back of a bench (or table which allows the foot to be clear of the ground). Take the paint can, dumbbell or other weight and attach it to the toe as before. Then, keeping the upper and lower leg still, *slowly* bend the foot upward. Hold for a count of 5, relax and repeat. Change the weight to the other foot and repeat.

Note: Holding on to the back of the

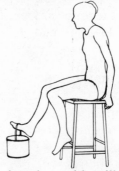

bench or table will help at first; this will become unnecessary later.

Repetitions: 5 each foot, increasing to 10

S19. Calf Raises

Stand erect, arms at sides, toes on the edge of a large book or shallow step. Bring the arms forward and raise the body upward until you are standing on your toes. Sink down again slowly. Rest and repeat.

Note: Keep the body upright; there is a tendency to lean forward. It is also of value to hold the position when half-way to the floor.

This is also an exercise which can be done on the floor without any book or ledge.

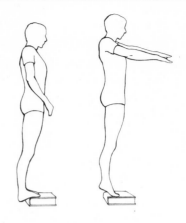

Repetitions: 5, increasing to 10

Strength Sports

The following sports are excellent for improving muscular strength:

General All-round Strength
Swimming
Wrestling
Weight Lifting
Nordic Skiing
Boxing
Rowing

Specific Muscle Strength
Canoeing—arms and upper body
Alpine Skiing—legs and lower body
Skating—legs and lower body
Cycling—legs

Weight Training

The most accepted and widely used strength-promoting method is weight training, which should not be confused with the sport of weight lifting.

Many types of apparatus can be found, from the ordinary barbell or dumbbell to more complicated machines, such as the Universal Gym, Nautilus and other designs. (The latter are found at fitness schools and gymnasiums, and as such are outside the scope of this book. However, many athletes are fortunate in having access to such apparatus and where weight-training facilities are available, it would be foolish not to make use of them.)

Under each sport, specific targets for training are mentioned, but weight training must never be practiced without proper supervision.

Exercises designed for building up pure "brute" strength involve considerable and increasing weights (high resistance) moved a comparatively few times (low repetition). These type of exercises tend to build up muscle power and muscle bulk and also generally harden the muscles. Exercises intended to increase muscle endurance involve comparatively low weights (low resistance) moved a large number of times (high repetition).

Always carry out a thorough warm-up (*see* pp. 40–41) before doing any weight lifting.

Weight training tends to shorten the muscles. Therefore after a training session, carry out gentle flexibility exercises to loosen the muscles, particularly the hamstring, lower back, arms and shoulders.

HEART AND LUNG EXERCISES

These exercises are designed to improve the performance of the heart (cardiovascular) and lung (respiratory) systems. They are extensively used as aids to general fitness and well-being, as well as having wide application for specific sports.

During strenuous exercise the body uses up oxygen at a very fast rate; if it is not replaced quickly enough or in large enough quantities, the body builds up an oxygen debt which soon leads to fatigue and exhaustion. Heart and lung exercises aim to correct this by increasing the body's capacity to take in oxygen, thus leading to greater stamina and endurance.

Ideally, carry out some form of heart and lung exercises for 20 minutes 3 times a week.

Jogging

As well as being a common activity and sport, jogging is an excellent heart and lung exercise, and many athletes carry out jogging as an alternative to other heart and lung pursuits, such as cycling or swimming. Jogging—both in place and around a court or a sports field—is a very good form of exercise as part of a warm-up routine or at the start of a training circuit for a specific sport. (For further details of jogging, see Part II).

Running in Place
(Spot Run, Running on the Spot)

This is not only an excellent heart and lung exercise, but a superb leg strengthener as well, especially for the hamstrings.

Raise the knees as high as you can and land on the balls of the feet.

Alternatively, raise each foot only 4 inches and jog in place.

Resistance Running

This can be in sand or other loose soil, up hills or across rough country. It, too, is an excellent leg strengthener (again for the hamstrings) and in addition improves eye/foot coordination.

Shuttle Runs

See p. 22.

Walking

An excellent heart and lung exercise, and probably the best way to gradually achieve fitness after a long lay-off or at the outset of an exercise regimen.

Walk purposefully, heel to toe, with a rolling gait. Breathe in deeply. Keep the back straight and the head up. Gradually lengthen the stride, swing the arms. Increase your walking distance and vary the terrain if you can.

Climbing Stairs

This is one of the best heart and lung exercises, and one of the easiest to find a suitable venue. Climb deliberately, placing the foot square on the step and rising slowly. Do not hurry. Set yourself a progressive target if you plan on using the same steps every day. Climbing 2 steps at a time is a useful variation.

Stadium steps: Frequent repetition in running up a stadium or other steps is an invaluable heart and lung exercise. It is also an excellent way of strengthening the leg muscles.

Ropework

The jump rope (or skipping rope) is one of the best heart and lung exercises there is and the benefits it offers are considerable. Not only does it improve stamina and endurance, but it helps keep the shoulders and arms flexible; strengthens the arm and leg muscles (as well as those in the calf and the ankle, if tiptoe jumping is adopted); fills out the neck, shoulders and chest; and is good for footwork and general agility.

Rope exercises are extremely strenuous, however. 10 minutes of rope work is equivalent to 20–30 minutes of jogging, so it is important to incorporate rest periods into your workout: jump until you are out of breath, then stop, rest for a few minutes and start again. At first you may be able to jump for only 20–30 seconds at a time. If you are overweight or over 30, or have a history of back pain, arthritis, heart trouble or sore feet, you should consult a doctor before beginning a rope program.

In any event, start with a low repetition and gradually build up. A few prior warm-up exercises are recommended, especially in cold weather.

Following are several simple jump rope exercises which athletes find useful in their training routines. Many variations on these are possible, and as you become more proficient with the rope you will probably want to devise your own. The most common variations involve jumping higher and turning the rope more than the usual once; carrying out intricate steps on touching the floor and before jumping again; and crossing the hands while turning the rope (*see* (3) *overleaf*).

Note: Make sure the rope is long enough. To test this, stand on it with both feet. The rope should reach the armpits on both sides.

1. Two-Footed Jumps. This is the basic jump-rope routine. Start with feet together, back straight and head erect, with the rope behind you. Bring the rope over the head and down in front of the feet. As it reaches them, jump up and let the rope pass under your feet. Bring the rope back behind you and repeat.

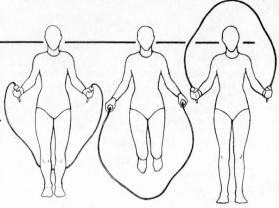

2. Running Step: With feet together, let the rope fall behind you, as shown. Swing rope over head and down in front of you. As it falls in front leap over it with the right foot leading. Land on the ball of the foot and balance with the left leg raised. Swing the rope over again and this time land on the left foot with the right leg raised. Repeat.

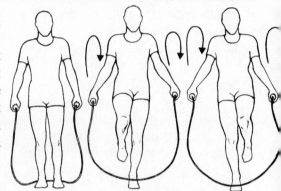

3. Cross-Over: As with Two-Footed Jumps, but as you jump cross the arms over as shown. Then carry out a normal two-foot jump and alternate with the Cross-Over. Repeat.

4. Side-to-Side: As for the Two-Footed Jumps, but jump to the right on landing, as shown, with the two feet together, and then to the left alternately. Repeat.

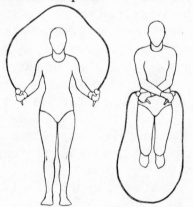

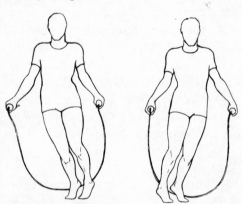

Other Stamina-Building Exercises

These are all strength exercises; however, if carried out at a fast rate, they are excellent stamina-building exercises as well.

S1. Push-Ups (Modified, for women and children)
S2. Pull-ups
S9. "Bicycling"

S12. Squat Thrusts (Burpees)
S16. Step-Ups
S17. Bench Jumps

Stamina-Building Sports

Cycling
Nordic Skiing
Swimming
Cross-Country and Long-Distance Running
Rowing, especially Sculling
Water Polo

Riding
Racquet Sports
Team Games (Football, Rugby, Soccer, Hockey, Lacrosse etc.)
Basketball
Scuba Diving
Boxing

Training Methods

RUNNING IS PROBABLY the best and certainly the most popular method of gaining heart and lung fitness. However, in recent years a number of different training methods utilizing running as a basis have been devised and found extremely valuable both as general and specific conditioners.

Fartlek Running (Swedish for "speed play")
This involves running (or swimming) long distances and varying the pace from fast to slow to fast again whenever the athlete feels the need. The attraction of this type of training is that it is entirely up to you to determine how fast to run. The disadvantage is that it requires a considerable amount of self-discipline to push yourself when you are really tired.

A Fartlek run might take the following form:

Jog for 300–400 yards
Sprint for 100 yards
Jog for 800 yards
Run fast for 200 yards
End with a 50-yard sprint

Interval Running
Interval running is a more disciplined version of Fartlek running, and is carried out to a strict schedule. A usual rule is that a slow interval should be 2–3 times as long as a fast effort. Then, as you attain a higher level of fitness, the slow intervals are shortened.

Here is a sample interval run:

Run 400 yards in 80 seconds
Jog for 100 yards
Run 400 yards
Repeat cycle several times.

Windsprints (Sprints)
Windsprints are an essential ingredient in conditioning for many sports, and are of great help in developing speed and getting the feel of increasing speed under control, which is essential in many team games.

In principle, windsprints comprise a gradual increase of speed for, say, 20 yards; a full speed sprint for 60 yards; then a slow-down for the last 20 yards, ending in a walk.

CIRCUIT TRAINING

None of the aforementioned training methods are really suitable for the casual or occasional athlete whose exercise time is brief and precious. Of greater benefit is circuit training, which is nothing more than a sequence of simple, non-time-consuming exercises designed to produce a balanced workout. These can be of a general conditioning nature, or designed specifically for individual sports, as shown in the home circuits under each sport in Part II.

Circuit training can be carried out in a gymnasium, out of doors (as many coaches prefer) or at home. For the casual or occasional sportsperson this is probably the best way to gain fitness for sport.

There are a number of guides to circuit training:

1. Sufficient exercises should be included to cover all muscle/body groups—a course of 8–10 is usually chosen.
2. Successive exercises should work on different parts of the body. In other words, don't choose two exercises for the arms immediately after each other.

Home Circuits

These can be worked out using either a single room or the whole house—the larger the area the greater the scope to make the circuit more interesting. Equipment required is minimal and improvisation possibilities are endless.

For Pull-Ups, a strong bar is a help—although the edge of the stairs will serve. A jump rope is useful, as are a couple of chairs, a few bricks or books, a plastic bag or two of sand, a tennis ball or simple rubber ball.

Important: It is not enough just to complete the circuit day after day. To gain benefit, exercise must be progressive. This can be done in several ways:

- By increasing the intensity
- By increasing the amount of time you spend exercising
- By increasing the number of repetitions
- By cutting down on the rest period between circuits

Duration and Repetitions: The figures shown in brackets are suggested as a possible starting number. For some people, even these low figures may be too much in some exercises, in which case you may initially prefer to start with a combination of less exhausting exercises from those listed earlier.

For others, the suggested repetitions are far below capacity, in which case when the entire circuit can comfortably be repeated 3 times as quickly without a break, increase the individual repetitions.

FOR GENERAL CONDITIONING
Circuit A
Preliminary warm-up. Jog on the spot for 1 minute. Rest 1 minute. Jog 1 minute.

S1.   Push-Ups or Modified Push-Ups (3)
S10. Bent-Leg Sit-Ups   (3)
F8.   Arm Flings   (8)
F2.   Trunk Twists   (6 each side)
S11. Half Squats   (4)
F4.   Neck Rolls   (6)
S16. Step-Ups   (4)
F6.   Wing Stretchers   (6)
S19. Calf Raises   (4)

Circuit B
Preliminary warm-up. Jog on the spot for 1 minute. Rest 1 minute, jog 1 minute.

F5.   Shoulder Shrugs   (6)
S4.   Hip Raises   (4)
S12. Squat Thrusts (Burpees)   (6)
F13. Leg Swings   (4 each side)
F3.   Alternate Toe Touches   (4 each side)
F11. The Lunge   (4 each side)
S10. Bent-Leg Sit-Ups   (3)
F14. Knee Pulls   (4 each side)

FITNESS TRAILS

Inspired by the Swiss exercise trails known as the Vita Parcours, fitness trails are increasingly coming into use in parks, playing fields and recreational areas. They consist of a series of "exercise stations" laid out along a jogging path or circuit, varying in length from anywhere from a quarter of a mile to several miles, and are designed to provide equipment (chin-up bars, ropes, hurdles, benches, logs, etc.), which the jogger can use as he or she rounds the circuit. The trails were developed to complement the cardiovascular benefits of running and jogging with exercises selected to increase strength in the abdomen, arms and shoulders as well as to improve body flexibility and balance.

For any jogger encountering one of these trails, there is a grave temptation—in the spirit of good health and enthusiasm that jogging brings—of hurling oneself into some pretty strenuous and taxing exercise routines before the body is ready for them. Be cautious. Don't try the more energetic exercises such as pull-ups, push-ups, sit-ups or rope climbing until you are ready for them; and when you think you are, approach any unaccustomed exercise on these circuits gradually and with caution. This is especially important for anyone over 40. Carry out 1 or 2 of each exercise first, and next time you pass do a few more.

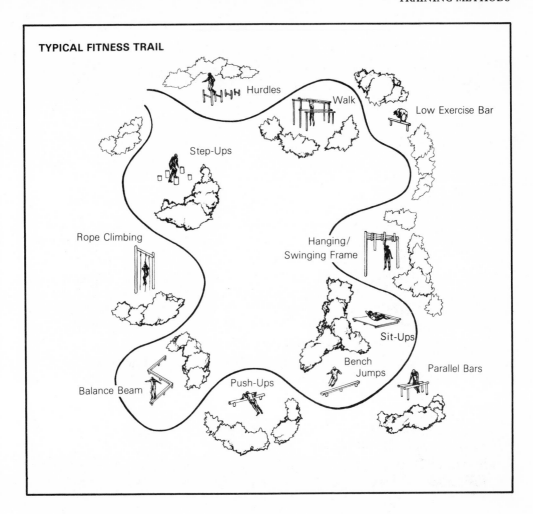

TYPICAL FITNESS TRAIL

Hurdles

Walk

Low Exercise Bar

Step-Ups

Rope Climbing

Hanging/
Swinging Frame

Sit-Ups

Bench
Jumps

Parallel Bars

Balance Beam

Push-Ups

Warming Up, Warming Down

YOU WILL NEVER SEE a serious athlete begin play without a preliminary warm-up. This may take the form of a gentle jog around the track or along the side of the playing field, or it may be the traditional rally before a tennis match or some calisthenics on the sidelines. The object is to loosen the body and warm and stretch the muscles, gradually introducing the heart and muscles to the forthcoming exercise, rather than subjecting them to the demands of sudden exertion before they are ready.

Inadequate warm-up can lead to pulled muscles, torn tendons, and a host of other strains and sprains. Limbering up improves the circulation of the blood and raises the body temperature, bringing the muscles into their most pliable condition. Increasingly, too, players and coaches alike are looking upon the warm-up period as having important psychological benefits in easing precompetition stress and keying the mind to the coming test.

The exercises listed below are for general warming-up purposes; warm-up routines associated with specific sports can be found in Part II, "Sport by Sport."

WARM-UP ROUTINE

The simplest warming-up exercise, and one that is used by athletes at all levels of expertise, is jogging in place for a few minutes. This is usually followed by simple stretching and flexing exercises to supple the body generally and to loosen those muscles most likely to be brought into play during the game. In racquet games, baseball, golf and many other sports, practice strokes help the limbering-up process. Also, in a number of sports, warming-up immediately prior to play includes passing, throwing, shooting or other actions associated with the game.

Warm-up should normally continue to the point of sweating, hence most players keep on their warm-up clothing (track suit, jacket or sweater, etc.)

until just before a game. In sports such as cricket, baseball and softball, warm-up should stop well before the point of sweating as long cold waits in the outfield can cause chills and muscle troubles. This is also true for cold-weather running, skiing (both Alpine and Nordic) and walking. In cold weather generally the warm-up should be more prolonged than when the weather is warm.

WARM-UP EXERCISES

Gentle jogging for a few minutes.

F1. Side Bends—hips and thighs
F2. Trunk Twists—trunk and neck
F3. Alternate Toe Touches—back, shoulders and arms
F7. Arm Circles—arms and upper body
F8. Arm Flings—arms, shoulders, wrists and hands
F10. The Reach—stomach, thigh and calf
F11. The Lunge—groin and thigh
F15. Calf Stretches—lower leg

This is just one of many possible routines. Exercise is a highly individual thing, and many players may prefer to vary the above according to their own preferences and requirements.

WARMING DOWN

In many ways warming down is almost as important as the preliminary warm-up. Warming down helps prevent muscle stiffness, and most players consider it an essential part of their routine.

After a game, match, race or practice session, walk and jog around for a few minutes. Do some Trunk Twists (F2) and Arm Circles (F7), and shake the wrists, hands and legs. Roll the neck and shoulders, and generally allow the body to cool down gradually. The object is to prevent the muscles from chilling, so it is advisable to put on a sweater, tracksuit top or jacket, etc., as soon as possible. Change out of sweaty clothes at the earliest opportunity.

WHAT SPORT?

Sport is the best and most interesting way to take exercise, at least in the eyes of many people. It does not have the monotony of running or walking, which, however beautiful the surroundings, can be a tedious occupation. Sport also provides competition and, on the whole, more challenge than that offered the walker or casual runner. And, although walking and running are liberating experiences, liberation is, or can be, more intense in sport.

But which sport? In Part II of this book the fitness aspects of nearly 60 different sports are covered, but the actual fitness benefits of these sports vary widely. Some time ago the International Committee on the Standardization of Physical Fitness Tests, whose findings were published as the *International Guide to Fitness and Health* by Leonard A. Larson and Herbert Mickleman (New York: Crown Publishers, Inc.) drew up a list of sports showing their effects on the three aspects of balanced fitness discussed in this book. Their adapted findings are below.

3 ratings are used: *** Great Effect ** Moderate Effect * Little or No Effect

	Mobility	Muscular Strength	General Endurance
ARCHERY	*	**	*
BADMINTON	**	**	**
BASEBALL	**	*	*
BASKETBALL	**	**	***
BOXING	*	***	***
CANOEING	*	***	**
CRICKET	**	*	*
CYCLING (Speed)	*	**	**
FENCING	***	**	*
FOOTBALL	**	**	**
GOLF	**	*	*
GYMNASTICS	**	**	*
HOCKEY (Field)	*	**	**
HOCKEY (Ice)	*	**	**
JUDO	**	**	*
KARATE	**	**	*
LACROSSE	**	**	**
RIDING	*	*	**
ROWING	*	*	***
RUGBY	**	**	**
RUNNING	*	**	***
SAILING	**	**	*
SCUBA	**	*	**
SKATING (Ice)	*	**	**
SKATING (Roller)	*	**	**
SKIING (Nordic)	**	***	***
SKIING (Alpine)	**	**	**
SOCCER	**	**	**
SQUASH	***	**	**
SURFING	**	**	*
SWIMMING	***	***	***
TABLE TENNIS	**	*	*
TENNIS	**	**	**
VOLLEYBALL	**	*	*
WALKING (Briskly 1 hour)	*	*	**
WATER POLO	**	**	***
WATER SKIING	**	**	**
WEIGHT LIFTING	*	***	*
WRESTLING	**	***	**

Diet

"A good diet—based on meat, milk, fish, poultry and eggs, whole grain cereals, legumes (peas and beans) and nuts, leafy green vegetables, and other vegetables and fruits—will meet the nutritional requirements of athletes."

L. JEAN BOGERT, *Nutrition and Physical Fitness*

THERE ARE AS MANY athlete's food fads and fancies as there are "popular" diets for the overweight. In some cases almost magical powers are ascribed to these foods and dietary supplements. Some seem to do good (although they are of apparently negligible nutritional value), principally perhaps because those who take them believe in them; few probably do harm if taken in moderation, provided common sense is practiced and there is some understanding of the form of balanced diet the body needs when being fully exercised.

Food is the fuel that powers the body and in order to function efficiently the body needs a number of substances to provide the raw material which is needed in the essential process of living. These are:

Carbohydrates (sugars and starches): Found in such foods as bread, potatoes, pasta, rice, grain and candy (sweets). These provide the primary source of quick energy that the body uses during exercise.

Proteins: Found in lean meat, eggs, fish, milk, cheese, peas and beans, and other pulses. They have no immediate energy value, but are essential to the long-term build-up of muscle and for many body functions.

Fats: The most concentrated source of energy in the diet. Weight for weight, they provide twice as much energy as carbohydrates. However, some fats—particularly the saturated fats, such as found in milk, cream, butter, lard and the fat in meat—are associated with high cholesterol levels in the blood, which in turn are connected with coronary heart disease. Thus an excessively fatty diet is unwise. It is best to cut down on fatty foods and make up bulk in the diet with more protein and carbohydrate.

Dietary Fiber: Principally roughage, fiber is a complex mixture of natural plant materials, most of which are not absorbed in the digestion process but affect the way other food substances are absorbed. A high-fiber diet is thought to protect against heart disease and diabetes. Best sources are cereals, wholemeal bread, potatoes, fruit and vegetables.

Vitamins: Vitamins are essential to good health, for they are vital catalysts for many body functions and are closely concerned with the chemical changes that take place within the body. There are well over one dozen vitamins, but all are found in adequate quantities in a normal, varied and well-balanced diet.

Minerals: In minute quantities, some minerals are essential for the well-being of the body. Iron, which is found in fish, liver, eggs and green vegetables, is an important constituent of the red bloods cells which carry the oxygen from the lungs and take it to all parts of the body. Calcium and phosphorus (which is found in the phosphate in milk) are necessary for bone and teeth production. Sodium (salt) is essential in the water-regulating processes of the body and is exuded in the form of sweat and urine—this is usually taken in the form of table salt and enough is commonly consumed in the daily diet. Potassium, magnesium and others are also necessary in varying amounts, but are usually found in sufficient quantities in a normal diet.

Water: The body comprises two-thirds water, and it serves as a diluting factor and helps transport waste products, as well as regulate body temperature. It is the main constituent of cell tissue and much is lost in sweat, urine and the breath. A balance has to be kept between water loss and water intake. If this is not maintained, the body becomes dehydrated—fortunately thirst is nature's warning device to prevent this from happening.

Even at rest the body needs at least 6 large glasses of water a day to function properly. In hot weather and when exercising, it needs a great deal more.

A good balanced diet is one which is as varied as possible and incorporates all the raw materials the body needs for nourishment. There are many books on general diets for the athlete, some of which are mentioned in the "Bibliography". However, to provide an easy guide, some years ago the US Department of Agriculture produced its Four-Food Plan based on the Recommended Daily Allowances (RDA) of nutrients as established by the US National Academy of Sciences. The plan divides the nutritional requirements of the body into 4 sections:

1. Milk and Milk Products
2. Meat, Fish and Shellfish, Poultry and Eggs.
3. Fruit and Vegetables
4. Bread and Cereals

2 large helpings of the first 2 groups and 4 large helpings of the last 2 every day will provide all the basic nutritional needs of the body.

Calories: All food contains potential energy which when eaten and acted upon will be released in the body. The unit of measurement used in calculating how much energy we get from the food we eat is the Calorie (which in the future will be replaced by the metric measurement known as Joules—4.2 Joules equals 1 Calorie).

To exist at all (that is, to carry on its basic functions such as breathing, digesting, sleeping, etc.), the body uses about 1,600 Calories a day.

On top of this figure should be added a work factor which varies according to the strenuousness of your occupation. A typist might require an extra 400 Calories a day, a carpenter or painter 1,400, an active outdoor worker 2,600 more.

In addition, any form of recreation or exercise adds to the energy requirement. The table below gives the Calories consumed per hour in a variety of different sports and activities.

CALORIES PER HOUR

Gentle Walking 175	Rollerskating 350
Walking Upstairs 200	Rowing (Easy) 300
Brisk Walking 435	Rowing (Sustained) 660–800
Hiking (40lb. pack) 300	Rowing (Sculling—Race) 840
Baseball 300	Running 900
Badminton (Competitive) 600	Skating (Recreational) 350
Basketball 600	Skating (Competitive) 450–780
Bicycling (Recreational) 250	Skiing—Alpine 300–500
Bicycling (9mph) 415	Skiing—Nordic 500–700
Canoeing (Paddling) 230	Squash 600–800
Canoeing (Competitive) 420	Swimming (Recreational) 300
Fencing 300	Table Tennis 450
Golf (No Cart) 300	Tennis (Competitive—singles) 600
Handball 600	Volleyball (Competitive) 600
Riding (Trotting) 415	Water Skiing 480

The daily calorific intake of many people, including every snack and break, is often far in excess of the body's basic requirements—even taking into account the Calories lost through normal day-to-day work and exercise. If Calorie consumption is excessive and not counterbalanced by that "burned" off through exercise and other bodily processes, the remainder will be stored in the form of fatty tissue. The body weight will rise and overweight will follow.

The desirable weight of men and women according to height and frame is shown in the table below, which was compiled by the Metropolitan Life Insurance Company.

DESIRABLE WEIGHTS (IN POUNDS)

Group	Height (with shoes on)	Small Frame	Medium Frame	Large Frame
Men (1-inch heels)	5' 2"	112–120	118–129	126–141
	5' 3"	115–123	121–133	129–144
	5' 4"	118–126	124–136	132–148
	5' 5"	121–129	127–139	135–152
	5' 6"	124–133	130–143	138–156
	5' 7"	128–137	134–147	142–161
	5' 8"	132–141	138–152	147–166
	5' 9"	136–145	142–156	151–170
	5' 10"	140–150	146–160	155–174
	5' 11"	144–154	150–165	159–179
	6' 0"	148–158	154–170	164–184
	6' 1"	152–162	158–175	168–189
	6' 2"	156–167	162–180	173–194
	6' 3"	160–171	167–185	178–199
	6' 4"	164–175	172–190	182–204
Women* (2-inch heels)	4' 10"	92–98	96–107	104–119
	4' 11"	94–101	98–110	106–122
	5' 0"	96–104	101–113	109–125
	5' 1"	99–107	104–116	112–128
	5' 2"	102–110	107–119	115–131
	5' 3"	105–113	110–122	118–134
	5' 4"	108–116	113–126	121–138
	5' 5"	111–119	116–130	125–142
	5' 6"	114–123	120–135	129–146
	5' 7"	118–127	124–139	133–150
	5' 8"	122–131	128–143	137–154
	5' 9"	126–135	132–147	141–158
	5' 10"	130–140	136–151	145–163
	5' 11"	134–144	140–155	149–168
	6' 0"	138–148	144–159	153–173

* For women between 18 and 25, subtract one pound for each year under 25.

These are average weights, and do not take into account those with unusually heavy bones or those who are particularly well-muscled, both of whom are technically overweight.

Another guide to weight levels is shown below.

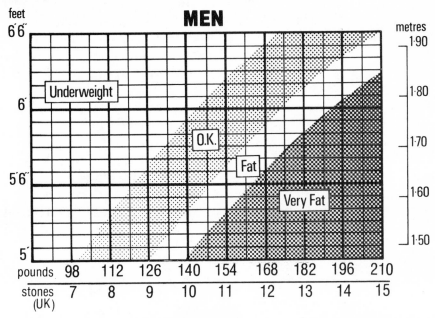

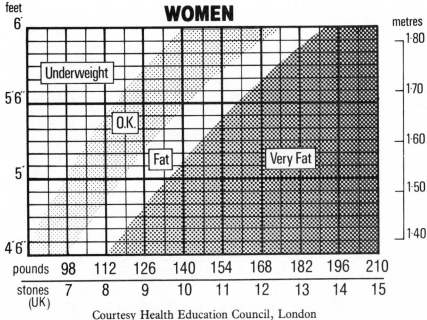

Courtesy Health Education Council, London

For those who are drastically overweight, obese in fact, Calorie intake is very important to monitor. Carrying extra weight demands that the heart works harder. Extra fat can lead to fatty substances—including cholesterol—being stored on the inside of the blood vessels. The more clogged the blood vessels become, the greater the likelihood of thrombosis and coronary heart disease. Mechanical trouble, brought about by the sheer physical effort involved in moving a heavy body around, could follow. This might include varicose veins, flat feet, arthritis and other joint trouble—particularly of the hip and knee. Also, general activity is cut down, and respiratory disease or kidney and liver complaints might ensue.

The process of weight increase is gradual. Every extra 3,000 Calories means an approximate increase of 1 pound in weight (or put another way, a 430 Calorie reduction each day will result in a 1 pound reduction in weight by the end of the week.) It is important to remember, however, that it took a long time to put on the extra poundage, so you must allow a reasonable time to lose it again. Nutrition and physiology experts alike are agreed that the best way—and not only for reasons of weight reduction—is to **eat less and exercise more.**

PRE-EXERCISE EATING

It is best to have an empty stomach when you run, walk, play a game or match, or exercise energetically, for food in the intestine can lead to stomach cramp, which is not only painful but will also impair performance.

Food takes a varying time to pass through the digestive system—and this can be prolonged by prematch tension—but the last pregame or prerun meal should be eaten at least 4 hours beforehand (some coaches advocate a liquid pregame meal, and this can be comfortably consumed as little as 2 hours before competition). However, many professional teams, because of the pregame stress factor, serve their last main meal 5–6 hours before a match. It is wise to avoid eating for at least 4 hours before taking part in sports involving abdomen contractions—such as wrestling, rowing or gymnastics.

A pregame meal should above all be easily digestible. It should be high in carbohydrate—to provide immediate energy. It should include fruit juice and ample fluid. It should be low in pure sugar, because a high level of sugar takes fluid from the body while being absorbed and may lead to dehydration, it also draws water into the stomach and can cause cramp. It should also be low in protein, as protein is not a source of immediate energy, and low in fat in view of the indigestible qualities of many fat products.

Avoid purely filling foods such as eggs, bacon or sausages; instead go for toast with jam or honey. Pancakes are a traditional pre-event meal before a number of competitions, but many athletes prefer to go on a complete fast before a game, race or match.

A sample pregame meal is:
Orange juice
Pancakes or toast with a small amount of butter, honey, syrup or jam
Fruit
Fruit juice
Milk, or tea with a small quantity of sugar

Another is:
Porridge
Bread and butter
Eggs
Coffee or milk

After the game
The principal need after exercise is to replace the considerable quantity of fluid that has been lost. The choice varies from athlete to athlete. Some prefer water, others fruit juice or soup, and most popular of all is beer.

Do not eat immediately after strenuous exercise, however, or you may become nauseous or get stomach cramp. Allow the body to cool down and slow down gradually to its normal state. Wait until you feel ready and wanting to eat—usually not less than 1 hour after a match.

PART II
Sport by Sport

How to use Part II

- A general description of its physical demands.
- A few notes on alternative or off-season activities that players and coaches have found useful for their own sport.
- Details of appropriate warm-up routines.
- Specific conditioning exercises, listed under Flexibility, Strength, and Heart and Lung (as in Part I).
- A home circuit of exercises, which can be carried out under your own roof and which are designed to aid specific fitness in each sport.
- A catalog of associated sports injuries, with an illustration to show specific trouble-spot sites and brief notes on prevention.

It should be noted that in some sports—particularly gymnastics , weight lifting, boxing, and track and field—conditioning is always carried out under the supervision of a coach or trainer. Thus for some sports you will find only the physical requirements, alternative sports and possible injuries listed. Your coach will have strong views about what, if any, specific conditioning exercises, warm-up routines and home-circuit training you should carry out to improve your fitness.

General Description: Some sports can be played at the recreational level without any prior fitness at all (for instance, riding, swimming and table tennis), but others cannot. This section analyzes the particular physical requirements of each sport, and what is needed in terms of heart and lung endurance, strength and flexibility.

Alternative Sports: Few other sports are actually detrimental to top performance in an athlete's primary sport, particularly at the weekend or part-time level, although some amateur players avoid those sports with a high likelihood of injury. Under each sport is a list of certain alternative games and sports that have been found to be of particular benefit in helping to develop a special skill or attribute, in strengthening or suppling a certain part of the body, or in building general all-round stamina.

Warm-Up: There are very few coaches or players who do not consider a thorough warm-up essential before play—partly to prevent strains and sprains to untuned, stiff muscles, and partly to help lower tension and get the mind in gear for the forthcoming match or game. Many sports have their own version of warm-up routine, which top players carry out as a matter of course.

Specific Fitness Exercises: To save the reader turning back to Part I, which gives a fairly exhaustive list of flexibility, strength, and heart and lung exercises, a list of these exercises of particular benefit to the athlete in each sport is given.

Home Circuit: Many sports lovers have neither the time nor the opportunity to exercise out of doors or in a gymnasium under the supervision of a coach or trainer. Accordingly, for most sports a home circuit has been included listing a sequence of 8–10 exercises that can be carried out under your own roof. The number of repetitions of these exercises is up to the individual. Initially, some exercises may be too strenuous or difficult for you, in which case you should turn back to Part I and choose an alternative. (Ropework, in particular, may not be a suitable activity for you if you are overweight or over 30, or if you suffer, or have ever suffered, from back pain, arthritis, heart trouble or sore feet.) When you get the "feel" of the circuit, you may prefer to devise your own from other exercises in Part I.

As a general guide, start with 2–3 repetitions of each exercise and go quickly through the circuit. When you have completed it, rest; then repeat. When you can complete the routine 3 times in succession and still carry on a conversation without puffing or panting, then—*and only then*—increase the repetitions a few at a time until you reach the optimum shown against each exercise in Part I. If there is any exercise which you cannot do comfortably, pass on to the next in the circuit, and next time substitute another less demanding one until you are more fit.

Sports Injuries: Each sport contains a list of injuries commonly associated with it as well as an illustration graphically depicting the likely trouble spots. (These illustrations show where injury *may* occur in a particular sport; they are by no means an indication of the quantity of injuries one can expect from a given sport.) It cannot be stressed too strongly that many of these injuries can be avoided altogether by specific sports conditioning and a really thorough warm-up before play. Details of prevention are also included.

Note: For more specific symptoms and treatment, the reader is referred to Part III, which provides more in-depth coverage of the more common sports injuries.

Jogging

JOGGING HAS COME TO BE accepted as one of the principal cures for modern-day living, and many people now jog as their only form of exercise. Medical opinions differ on the relative values and dangers of jogging, but there is universal agreement that jogging should be taken easily at first (especially if you are overweight or unaccustomed to exercise). Jogging should be looked upon as an exacting form of recreation, and as such should only be practiced after initial fitness tests (*see* Part I). Rather than plunge straight into jogging, the logical and sensible progression is to start off with a walking program, then alternate between walking and jogging until you feel ready to jog full time. Even then take it easy and build up distance gradually.

Specific fitness for jogging involves a degree of stamina, and some strength and flexibility in the upper body, leg and arms.

Warm-Up: Very few joggers do any warming-up before jogging as they consider the exercise they are about to take as warm-up enough. If they did limber up, though, the incidence of jogging injuries—sore or pulled muscles, etc.—would be very much less.

A good routine is to spend 1–2 minutes jogging on the spot and then carry out a few flexibility exercises, with emphasis on the back, body, shoulder, arms, and upper and lower legs. These might include:

F1. Side Bends—hips and thighs
F2. Trunk Twists—trunk and neck
F3. Alternate Toe Touches—back, shoulders and arms
F9. Wrist Shakes—wrists and hands
F10. The Reach—stomach, thighs and calf
F13. Leg Swings—thighs

BAD-WEATHER HOME CIRCUIT

If the weather is unsuitable for jogging, the frustrated jogger should try a home circuit. This might include:

Preliminary Warm-Up
Jogging on the spot
F1.   Side Bends
S1.   Modified Push-Ups
F7.   Arm Circles
S11. Half Squats
F9.   Wrist Shakes
S18. Shin Strengtheners
F10. The Reach
F13. Leg Swings

JOGGING INJURIES

Jogging injuries are almost all to the lower limbs, with the exception of injuries due to accidental falls or collisions which might hurt any part of the body.

Choose loose, comfortable clothing; jogging or track suits are ideal, but not essential. The important thing is for you to be warm enough in winter, cool enough in summer, and comfortable whenever you jog. Plastic clothing is not advisable as it will make you sweat excessively and cause the body temperature to rise which, in extreme cases, could lead to heat exhaustion or heat stroke (*see* Part III). Footwear should be comfortable with good soles, good heel and sole support, and soft, pliable tops. It is inadvisable to wear thin-soled shoes.

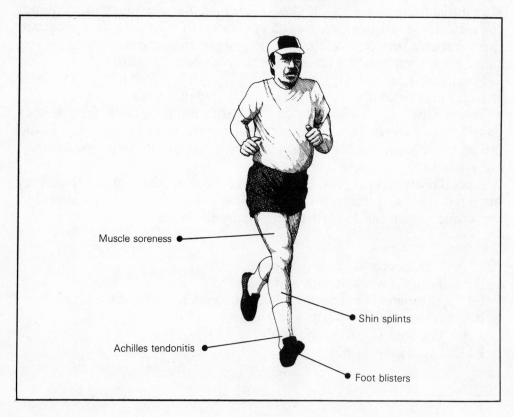

Muscle soreness

Shin splints

Achilles tendonitis

Foot blisters

Blisters: A common jogging complaint. Use alcohol or some other skin-hardening agent on the feet before beginning a jogging program.

Other jogging foot ailments are *shin splints* and *Achilles tendonitis*. Stretching and strengthening exercises for the lower leg should render these less likely. (There injuries are all more thoroughly covered in Part III.)

Sore muscles are a characteristic of doing any unaccustomed exercise. A hot bath or shower immediately after your run, with some stretching and flexing under water, should do much to ease potential discomfort and prevent stiffness the following day.

If you have any illness or sickness, leave off jogging until the condition has worn off.

Cycling

CYCLING AS A RECREATIONAL exercise is regarded as one of the finest stamina builders. As a sport it is one of the most exacting, calling on a very high degree of all-round fitness.

Specifically, cycling demands great heart and lung endurance; strength, especially in the body and legs; and flexibility, particularly in the lower body.

Alternative Sports: Alternative or off-season sports include racquet games, especially squash and badminton. Swimming and running are good stamina builders. Best of all, when the equipment is available, is stationary cycle training.

Warm-Up: This should include gentle flexibility exercises, as well as "Bicycling" (S9—*see* p. 27). Then do some short sprints and longer distance workouts in order to gradually ease the muscles involved in cycling.

CYCLING FITNESS EXERCISES
Flexibility
F1. Side Bends—hips and thighs
F2. Trunk Twists—trunk and neck
F3. Alternate Toe Touches—back, shoulders and arms
F7. Arm Circles—arms and upper body
F10. The Reach—stomach, thigh and calf
F12. Hurdles—groin and thigh
F15. Calf Stretches—lower leg

Strength
S1. Push-Ups or Modified Push-Ups—body
S2. Pull-Ups—arms and shoulders
S10. Bent-Leg Sit-Ups—abdomen
S15. Leg Raises—upper leg
S16. Step-Ups—upper leg
S19. Calf Raises—lower leg

In addition, weight training under supervision, especially for body and legs.

Heart and Lung
Running, including Fartlek and inter-
val training
Swimming
Ropework

HOME CIRCUIT
Jogging on the spot
Ropework, if appropriate; otherwise
jogging
S1. Push-Ups or Modified Push-Ups
F2. Trunk Twists
F12. Hurdles
S10. Bent-Leg Sit-Ups
S16. Step-Ups
F3. Alternate Toe Touches
S2. Pull-Ups
F1. Side Bends

CYCLING INJURIES
Blisters (hands): Especially common
with distance riders, and often due to a
bad position.

Chafing: This usually occurs on the
bottom and the upper leg, and is commonly due to wearing poorly made
shorts. The ideal material is wool, with
chamois leather lining. If the seams are
rough or in the wrong place, or the
leather is coarse, chafing will occur.
Pure lanolin (medical, not cosmetic) or
other soothing cream will clear this up
quickly, and is also a useful preventative. Synthetic linings for shorts are
available in many places and some seem
effective in eliminating chafing.

Toe Chafing: A condition mainly

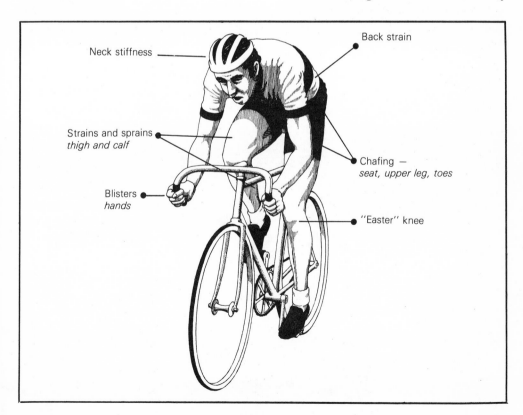

Neck stiffness

Back strain

Strains and sprains
thigh and calf

Chafing —
seat, upper leg, toes

Blisters
hands

"Easter" knee

affecting the very long distance or touring cyclist. It is caused either by ill-fitting toe clips or shoes.

"Easter Knees": A colloquial name for a cycling condition that is common at the start of the season, hence its nickname. It is caused by riding too fast too early. Anatomically, it is a pulled muscle just below the knee joint. It should be treated as other muscle pulls (*see* Part III).

Back Strain: Particularly of the lower back. This is usually due to a faulty cycling position. If mild, a hot bath or shower and gentle flexing exercises under water should ease the discomfort considerably. If more severe, it is best to consult a doctor. If persistent but mild, consult a cycling coach about your riding style.

Sprains and Strains: Especially of the thighs and calves. This is almost always due to either riding too fast too early, or because of inadequate warm-up before a race. Strength and flexibility exercises should do much to prevent this.

Falls: Falls are responsible for the most severe cycling injuries. These can vary from mild bruising, to cuts, abrasions and fractures (especially of the collarbone) and even concussions.

Neck Stiffness: This is another early-season complaint brought about by wearing too much clothing around the neck. A single scarf should be sufficient in even the coldest weather; some cyclists prefer to wear none at all.

Riding

RIDING IS RECOGNIZED as one of the finest all-round sports and recreations. Casual riding can be enjoyed with little or no prior fitness. In fact, it is considered an excellent therapy for the disabled and for the rehabilitation of the injured. If the rider takes part in jumping, eventing or fox hunting, a degree of physical fitness is definitely required.

Specifically, a high standard of heart and lung endurance is required. Great strength is not needed under modern teaching, but flexibility is important, particularly in the wrists and hands, hips, knees and ankles. Relaxation of the whole body is crucial to successful riding, as tension in the rider is communicated immediately to the horse and can have a disastrous effect on the essential harmony between rider and mount.

Alternative Sports: Top-class riders find racquet sports, swimming and running useful all-around sports for riding. Judo, aikido and wrestling are invaluable for helping the rider learn how to fall correctly—most serious riding injuries are due to falls.

Warm-Up: Flexibility exercises are recommended before you mount, but most riders tend to do their limbering up on the back of the horse. These include:

F4. Neck Rolls—neck
F5. Shoulder Shrug—shoulders
F7. Arm Circles—arms and upper body
F13. Leg Swings—upper legs

These exercises can also be carried out on foot.

RIDING FITNESS EXERCISES
Flexibility

F1. Side Bends—hips and thighs
F2. Trunk Twists—trunk and neck
F4. Neck Rolls—neck
F5. Shoulder Shrugs—shoulders
F7. Arm Circles—arms, upper body
F9. Wrist Shakes—wrists and hands
F11. The Lunge—groin and thighs
F13. Leg Swings—upper leg

Strength

S4. Hip Raises—arms and shoulders
S6. Tennis Ball Squeeze—wrists and hands
S8. Fingertip Hip Raise—fingers
S10. Bent-Leg Sit-Up—abdomen
S17. Bench Jumps—upper leg

Heart and Lung

Running   Swimming
Jogging   Ropework

HOME CIRCUIT

Preliminary warm-up
Ropework, if appropriate; otherwise jogging
F5. Shoulder Shrugs
F13. Leg Swings
F7. Arm Circles
S17. Bench Jumps
F4. Neck Rolls

F9. Wrist Shakes
S10. Bent-Leg Sit-Ups
F11. The Lunge

RIDING INJURIES

Some riding injuries occur on the horse, but by far the more serious ones happen in falling. In addition, riders are sometimes injured by being kicked by another horse or, after a fall, if their own mount rolls over on them. This can result in fractured legs or ankles, or other more serious injuries.

Blisters—Inside Knee: Caused by loose, badly fitting trouser legs which rub between the rider's leg and the saddle. If severe, it may be necessary to stop riding until the blisters clear up. In most cases, however, strapping or an elastic bandage will provide the necessary protection. **Hands:** Due to the reins

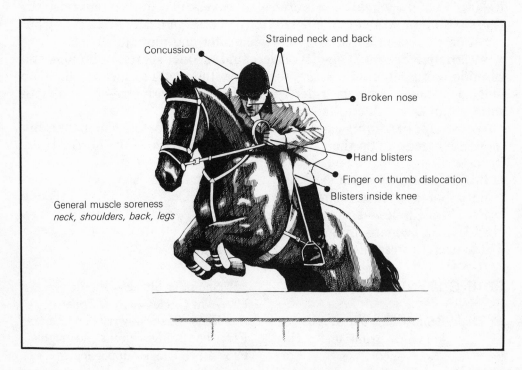

Concussion

Strained neck and back

Broken nose

Hand blisters

Finger or thumb dislocation

Blisters inside knee

General muscle soreness
neck, shoulders, back, legs

rubbing on the soft skin of the hands. It is advisable to wear riding gloves, which also help prevent the reins from slipping if the hands become sweaty or the rider is caught in the rain.

General Muscle Soreness: Particularly in neck, shoulders, back and legs. commonly due to the effect of unaccustomed activity. The stiffness and soreness will wear off after a few days. A hot bath or shower (during which you should flex and manipulate the muscles under the water), sauna, massage or swimming in a heated pool are all benficial. Best of all is further riding to get the muscles into riding trim.

Broken Nose: This is generally due to falls or to the horse tossing up his head and catching the rider in the face, which can also cause cut lips and broken teeth. It is first necessary to stop any bleeding from the nose. Dismount, and either ask someone to hold your horse or tie it up. Sit down on the ground and lean forward. Spit out any blood; do not swallow it. Squeeze nose with thumb and forefinger for 3–6 minutes. If cold water is available—a stream or pond—soak a handkerchief or rag and apply it to the back of the neck and over the nose (ice is better still, if available). The angle of the nose will show if it is broken; you should see a doctor as soon as you can to have it reset.

The only prevention is general alertness and correct riding posture and jumping technique.

Strains and Sprains of Neck and Back: These are often caused by a restless or bucking horse which jars the rider. Apply ice to the affected area, and rest. If more severe, it is advisable to see a doctor, as the injury may require extensive treatment.

Finger or Thumb Dislocations: This frequently occurs in jumping, when the rider's hands are jerked on to the horse's neck. Make yourself—or the victim—as comfortable as possible until a doctor can see the injury. Temporary strapping to the next finger may save pain from jarring.

Concussion: This is a common—and potentially very serious—riding injury usually caused by a fall. For symptoms and treatment, *see* Part III.

A correctly fitting hard riding hat is essential protection. It is now believed that the former custom of wearing a harness chinstrap with a peaked riding hat can lead to a broken neck if the hat is jerked upwards in a fall. Therefore, no chinstrap should be worn if the hat is peaked, and the hat should fit so well that it will not come off in a fall—very few borrowed riding hats fulfil that condition.

Event riders and jockeys wear detachable and flexible peaks when riding.

Other severe riding injuries can be caused when the rider catches a foot in the stirrup when falling and is dragged along by a bolting horse. This can be largely prevented by wearing riding boots or shoes with a heel; flat-soled shoes are highly dangerous as the foot can slip all the way through the stirrup thus trapping the leg.

Gymnastics

GYMNASTICS IS PROBABLY the most testing and demanding of all sports, and one requiring the highest level of all-round physical ability. The sport calls for a very high level of general fitness, considerable stamina, various specific strengths, body suppleness, balance, agility, rhythm and supreme body control and coordination—not to mention whole-hearted dedication.

A high standard of general conditioning is vital for building confidence and promoting safety on the apparatus. More specifically, it demands a very high level of heart and lung endurance; strength, particularly in the body as well as in the arms and legs; and all-round suppleness.

Alternative Sports: Jogging and walking as well as ropework are all good for building general stamina. Rope climbing is a useful aid to strength training. Team games, such as soccer and basketball, and racquet sports such as squash and badminton are good for improving general agility. Modern dance and ballet are invaluable in improving suppleness and rhythm.

GYMNASTICS INJURIES

Ankle injuries: A common occurrence in gymnastics, they are often due to landing incorrectly. Proper landing is crucial to successful and injury-free gymnastics. Flexibility and strength exercises will do much to lessen or minimize such injuries.

Lower back pain: This can also result from many of the exercises and routines in gymnastics. A full program of flexibility and strengthening exercises is essential in gymnastics conditioning, as is a thorough warm-up before a training session or competition.

Blisters and calluses: These are apt to occur and can be a severe handicap. It is advisable to harden the hands with alcohol or other skin-hardening agents.

General sprains and strains: These can occur to many parts of the body in such an exacting sport as gymnastics. The only real preventative is a complete program of flexibility and strength exercises and a thorough warm-up before a workout or competition.

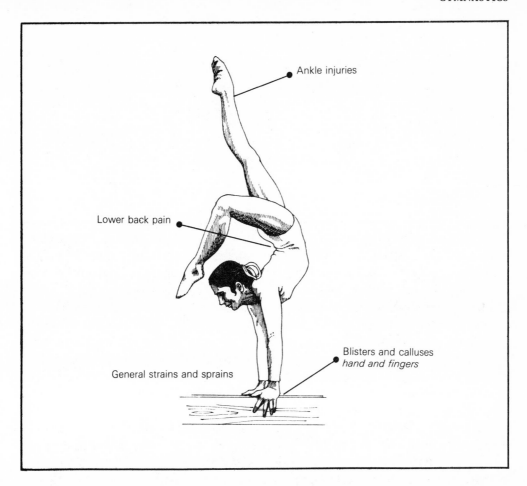

Ankle injuries

Lower back pain

Blisters and calluses
hand and fingers

General strains and sprains

Other injuries such as bruising, cuts, abrasions and fractures can occur if a gymnast falls or strikes the apparatus or if a piece of equipment breaks while being used. It is essential that equipment be properly looked after. It should also be thoroughly checked out from time to time.

Weight Lifting

WEIGHT LIFTING is an Olympic sport which calls for considerably more than sheer strength. Among other things, it demands good reflexes, perfect body coordination, utter dedication and a high level of courage. It should not be taken up too young and most countries have a minimum age of 12–13 before competitive weight lifting is permitted, although weight training is encouraged at a much earlier age.

Specifically, weight lifting requires a reasonable degree of heart and lung endurance, for although individual lifts may take no more than a few seconds, a contest can last for hours; strength, particularly in the body, shoulders, arms, wrists and legs; and flexibility in the body, shoulders and legs, knees and ankles.

Alternative Sports: Running, particularly cross-country and sprinting, are good stamina builders during the off-season period; the latter is also useful in developing reaction speed. Squash, for its capacity to give an intense workout in a short time, and soccer or football are other useful alternatives. Gymnastics is excellent for building all-round suppleness.

Warm-Up: This is extremely important in a sport that places such supreme strain on the muscles. It usually takes the form of flexibility exercises followed by weight-lifting practice, to within 10 pounds of the ultimate weight.

Warm-Down: The warm-down after practice or competition is as important as the preliminary warm-up and should comprise some jogging followed by stretching exercises.

WEIGHT-LIFTING FITNESS EXERCISES

Training for weight-lifting contests is often divided into three parts:

1. An initial period designed to promote overall fitness which incorporates flexibility, strength, and heart and lung exercises, as well as specific weight-lifting conditioning.
2. A period devoted to power development, using intensive weight training to build up muscle volume and strength.
3. A final period to develop lifting skills and techniques.

Suitable exercises for the initial period are:

Flexibility

F2. Trunk Twists—trunk and neck
F3. Alternate Toe Touches—back, shoulders and arms
F6. Wing Stretchers—shoulders
F8. Arm Flings—arms and upper body
F11. The Lunge—groin and thighs
F12. Hurdles—groin and thighs
F14. Knee Pulls—lower legs
F15. Calf Stretches—lower legs

Strength

S1. Push-Ups—body
S2. Pull-Ups—arms and shoulders
S5. Broomstick Rolls—wrists and hands
S10. Bent-Leg Sit-Ups—abdomen

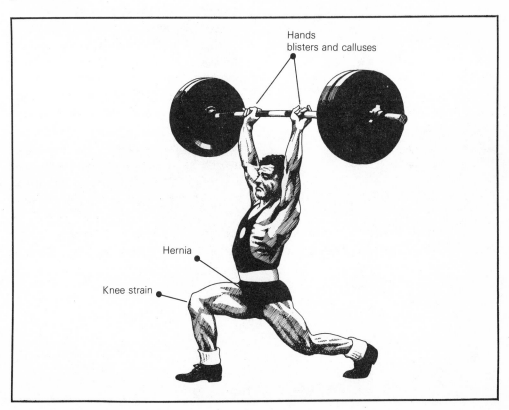

Hands
blisters and calluses

Hernia

Knee strain

S11. Half Squats—thighs
S12. Squat Thrusts—thighs
S16. Step-Ups—upper legs
S17. Bench Jumps—upper legs
S19. Calf Raises—lower legs

In addition, specific weight training under supervision.

Heart and Lung
Running, particularly Fartlek and interval training, uphill and sandhill work; shuttle runs and sprints for improving speed.
Ropework
Swimming

HOME CIRCUIT
Preliminary warm-up
Jogging on the spot
Ropework
S1. Push-Ups
F2. Trunk Twists
F12. Hurdles
S10. Bent-Leg Sit-Ups
S16. Step-Ups
F3. Alternate Toe Touches
S2. Pull-Ups
S12. Squat Thrusts

WEIGHT-LIFTING INJURIES
The first rule of weight lifting is that lifting should *always* be done with a straight back. Providing this advice is followed, injuries in the sport are comparatively few.

Blisters and Calluses: These are frequent and can be a handicap, so hand-hardening well before the season starts is essential.

Knee Strain: This may be caused by the cumulative effect of weight lifting over many years—or it may occur suddenly, often as a result of bad technique. Extensive flexibility and strengthening exercises in the conditioning program combined with a really thorough warm-up before a training session or match should do much to lessen the likelihood of knee strain.

Hernias or Ruptures: This is a small amount of gut or fat that is pushed up through the lower edge of the abdomen muscles by sudden exertion or even a spasm of coughing. It can occur to even the fittest athlete, but those with weak abdominal muscles are most vulnerable. The principal symptom is a swelling in the groin, small at first but becoming larger; it may or may not be accompanied by pain. Treatment may involve an operation or wearing a truss. Developing the abdominal muscles is the best way of preventing a rupture. Avoid making sudden strains on the abdomen and ensure when lifting that the back is perfectly straight.

Archery

ARCHERY AS A RECREATION requires little or no prior fitness. Competition archery, on the other hand, calls for both good physical conditioning and a high degree of body control allied with a good posture and a great deal of mental discipline.

Target archery demands a fair level of heart and lung endurance; strength in the upper body and arms, to provide enough pulling power to draw the modern bow; and flexibility in the neck, shoulders, upper and lower back, wrists and fingers.

Field archery, in addition to target archery's attributes, requires considerable stamina and rather more strength in the shoulders as well as in the legs. Above all, it demands great flexibility of the spine in order to be able to shoot up and downhill and from a variety of different postures.

Alternative Sports: Running, swimming, jogging and cycling are all good for general stamina building, but walking is best. Racquet sports, such as squash and badminton, are excellent, as are basketball and volleyball, both of which involve a lot of back muscle work as well as wrist flexibility. Gymnastics (for general suppleness), yoga and martial arts such as aikido are also valuable.

Warm-Up: Carry out flexibility exercises, especially for the back, neck and shoulders. It is important to lower tension as much as possible, partly for reasons of performance, partly to lessen the chance of muscle strain.

ARCHERY FITNESS EXERCISES
Flexibility

F1. Side Bends—hips and thighs

F2. Trunk Twists—trunk and neck

F3. Alternate Toe Touches—back, shoulders and arms

F4. Neck Rolls—neck

F6. Wing Stretchers—shoulders

F8. Arm Flings—arms, upper body

F9. Wrist Shakes—wrists and hands

Strength

S1. Push-Ups or Modified
Push-Ups—body

S2. Pull-Ups—arms and shoulders

S5. Broomstick Rolls—wrists and hands

S6. Tennis Ball Squeeze—wrists and hands

S8. Fingertip Hip Raises—fingers

Heart and Lung

Running
Swimming
Cycling
Ropework
Walking

Walking is probably the best heart and lung exercise for the archer. The average sedentary life, especially sitting at an office desk, leads to round shoulders and poor posture, both of which are disastrous for the archer. When walking, "walk tall," forcing shoulders back and breathing in deeply.

HOME CIRCUIT

Preliminary Warm-Up
Jogging on the spot
Ropework if appropriate, otherwise jogging
F4. Neck Rolls

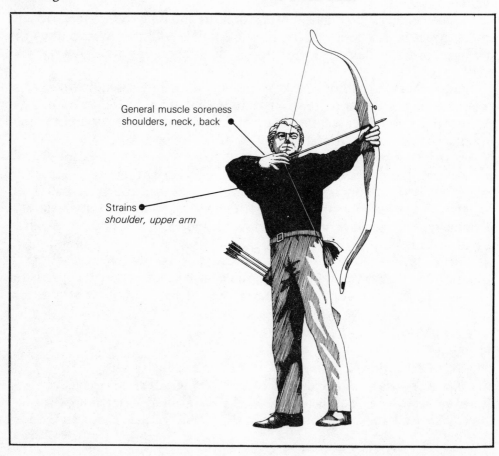

General muscle soreness
shoulders, neck, back

Strains
shoulder, upper arm

S1. Push-Ups or Modified Push-Ups
F2. Trunk Twists
S8. Fingertip Hip Raises
F3. Alternate Toe Touches
S2. Pull-Ups
F8. Arm Flings
F1. Side Bends

ARCHERY INJURIES

Archery is an almost injury-free sport, and those few aches and pains that occur can be almost wholly prevented by proper conditioning and a thorough warm-up.

Muscle Soreness: Particularly to the shoulders, neck and back. This soon wears off and is usually due to a combination of poor conditioning and tension, especially in the novice. A hot shower or bath, and gentle muscle flexing under water works wonders.

Strains: Particularly to the shoulder and the upper arm. These are principally due to poor conditioning, but your technique may also be at fault, so see a coach for advice. Equally, your bow may be too strong.

Field archers are liable to twist ankles or otherwise injure themselves in falls while crossing rough country. Shoes or boots with good studs are essential to prevent slipping, golfing shoes are ideal. As competitions are liable to go on for many hours, away from a clubhouse or other form of proper shelter, it is always advisable to carry some form of waterproof covering or coat.

Baseball and Softball

BASEBALL AND SOFTBALL can be enjoyed with no conditioning at all, but to play either game to the full at a competitive level requires a high standard of general fitness, and there is little doubt that sound conditioning brings confidence as well as prevents against strains and sprains.

Specifically, baseball and softball players need a high degree of heart and lung endurance as well as the ability to employ explosive bursts of speed over short distances.

Batting requires strength in the upper body and wrists.

Pitching and throwing demands strength in the shoulders, back, arms and legs, as well as flexibility in the back, arm and wrists.

Alternative Sports: Running, jogging, swimming and cycling are all good for stamina building. Racquet sports such as squash and badminton, basketball and golf—all of which require a degree of flexibility and good hand/eye coordination—are useful off-season or alternative sports.

Warm-Up: Most players jog for a while and then carry out flexibility exercises, with emphasis on back, arms, wrists and legs. Do practice swings with a weighted bat. Pitchers should exercise the pitching arm in preparation for the immediate and explosive effort they will have to exert from the outset. Start with limited-range-of-motion exercises and extend to full-range ones.

BASEBALL AND SOFTBALL FITNESS EXERCISES

Flexibility

F1. Side Bends—hips and thighs
F2. Trunk Twists—trunk and neck
F3. Alternate Toe Touches—back, shoulders and arms
F7. Arm Circles—arms and upper trunk
F10. The Reach—stomach, thighs and calves
F11. The Lunge—groin and thighs
F12. Hurdles—groin and thighs
F15. Calf Stretches—lower legs

Strength

S1. Push-Ups or Modified Push-Ups—body

S2. Pull-Ups—arms and shoulders
S7. Fingertip Push-Ups—fingers
S8. Fingertip Hip Raises—fingers
S10. Bent-Leg Sit-Ups—abdomen
S12. Squat Thrusts—thighs
S13. Sprinters—thighs
S17. Bench Jumps—upper legs
S19. Calf Raises—lower legs

In addition, weight training under supervision. Low-resistance, high-repetition exercises especially for body, arms and wrists.

Heart and Lung

Running, particularly Fartlek and interval training; shuttle runs and sprints are also excellent (40 yards maximum distance, with a lot of work at 15–20 yards)
Jogging
Cycling

HOME CIRCUIT

Ropework, if appropriate; otherwise jogging
S1. Push-Ups or Modified Push-Ups
F2. Trunk Twists
F12. Hurdles
S10. Bent-Leg Sit-Ups
F3. Alternate Toe Touches
S2. Pull-Ups
S17. Bench Jumps
S12. Squat Thrusts
S8. Fingertip Hip Raises

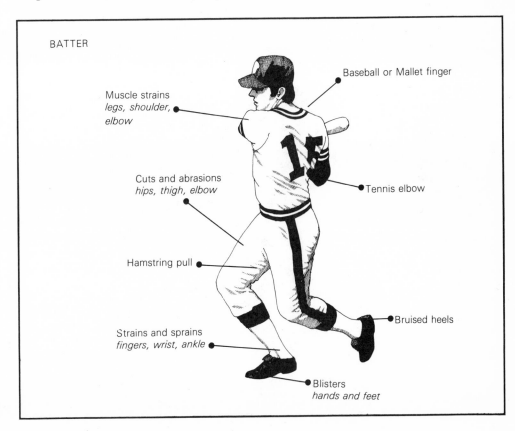

BATTER

Muscle strains
legs, shoulder, elbow

Baseball or Mallet finger

Cuts and abrasions
hips, thigh, elbow

Tennis elbow

Hamstring pull

Strains and sprains
fingers, wrist, ankle

Bruised heels

Blisters
hands and feet

BASEBALL AND SOFTBALL INJURIES

Blisters (Hands, occasionally Feet):
Hand blisters may develop in both baseball and softball from gripping the bat too hard and from throwing. Foot blisters are common, particularly at the start of the season before the feet are fully hardened. Use either alcohol or a skin-hardening agent to harden both hands and feet.

Cuts and Abrasions: These frequently occur as a result of sliding into base, and are especially common to the hips, thighs and elbows. Spike cuts are often much deeper than they first appear and it is extremely important that they be thoroughly cleansed with soap and water to eliminate any chance of infection. If really deep, they may well need stitching, so consult a doctor.

Strains and Sprains: These are quite common in baseball and softball. Most vulnerable are the fingers, wrists and ankles, particularly when sliding into base. (Bruised heels can also result.)

General Muscle Strains: These occur in the legs, shoulders and inner side of the elbow. These can often lead to some swelling as well as considerable pain.

Hamstring Pulls: Base runners and outfielders are particularly vulnerable. Like all strains and sprains they can

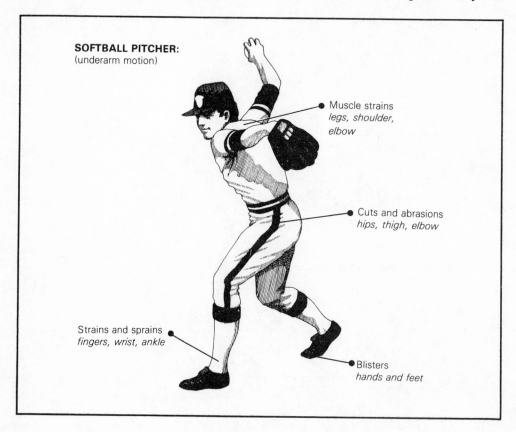

SOFTBALL PITCHER:
(underarm motion)

Muscle strains
legs, shoulder, elbow

Cuts and abrasions
hips, thigh, elbow

Strains and sprains
fingers, wrist, ankle

Blisters
hands and feet

largely be prevented by carrying out flexibility and strengthening exercises during conditioning and a really thorough warm-up before a game.

Mallet or Baseball Finger: This is caused by failing to catch the ball cleanly. As a result it strikes the end of the finger and, in addition to causing great pain and swelling, it breaks the tendon holding up the top joint. In consequence the fingertip droops. Treatment may involve splinting for up to 6 weeks.

Tennis Elbow: This occasionally afflicts batters—particularly long-distance hitters who fail to follow through properly—and pitchers. For treatment and some ways to ease the pain, *see* Tennis p. 129.

Strain of the Lumbar Muscles (Back): Pitchers are particularly prone here. Strength and flexibility exercises should do much to avoid this complaint. Warm-up is absolutely crucial to the pitcher and must be thorough.

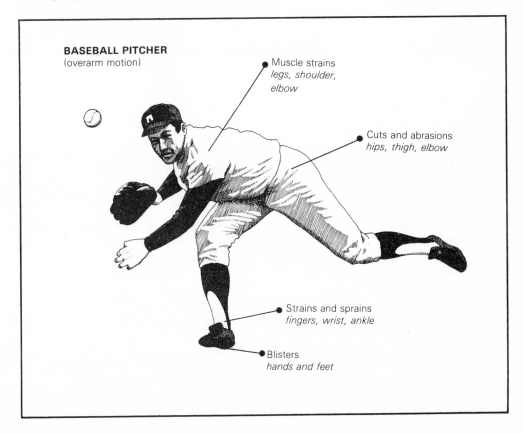

BASEBALL PITCHER
(overarm motion)

Muscle strains
legs, shoulder, elbow

Cuts and abrasions
hips, thigh, elbow

Strains and sprains
fingers, wrist, ankle

Blisters
hands and feet

Cricket

CRICKET IS A SPORT in which the fitness aspect is almost totally neglected until a player nears the highest levels. The physical demands of the sport can be considerable, however. A fieldsman, after long and possibly cold hours in the field, is called upon for sudden explosive bursts of effort often involving turning, acceleration and quick stops. A batsman needs considerable reserves of stamina in a long innings, and at any time may be required to make a sudden start-stop or hurried change of direction. A fast bowler expends a large amount of energy and places considerable strain on his whole body, particularly the upper half. A wicket keeper remains in a semi-crouched position for long periods, and from this awkward stance is required to exert spring and explosive effort at any time. Over all, the risks are high in any game played with a hard ball on an unyielding, often rough or slippery, surface.

Specifically, a batsman requires a high standard of general fitness; excellent coordination of hand and eye; a degree of strength, particularly in back, shoulders, forearms and wrists; and flexibility in trunk, shoulders, elbows, wrists and knees.

A fieldsman needs all-round fitness. A close fieldsman must have great flexibility, especially in back, trunk, shoulders and legs.

A fast bowler requires a very high degree of general fitness; strength, above all in trunk, abdomen, shoulders, arms and legs; and flexibility in the upper body, arms, wrists and fingers.

A slow bowler requires the same degree of general fitness, but depends less on strength. He does, however, require a very high degree of flexibility in arms, wrists and fingers.

A wicket keeper principally requires trunk flexibility and strength in the neck, back and legs, particularly in the quadriceps and hamstring muscles.

Alternative Sports: Racquet sports such as tennis, badminton, squash and table tennis are excellent alternative sports for improving hand/eye coordination. Volleyball and basketball are also popular. Running, especially sprinting, is good for improving stamina. Many players find great relaxation in golf; others prefer soccer or rugby. Top-class players aim to take some form of major exercise at least once a week in the winter months.

Warm-Up: The warm-up in cricket is usually rather neglected, but it is of particular importance to close fieldsmen, batsmen just before they open their innings and bowlers. Jogging and gentle stretching and flexing exercises are advisable, but it is important in a game as protracted as cricket *not* to warm up to the point of sweating.

CRICKET FITNESS EXERCISES

Flexibility

F2. Trunk Twists—trunk and neck

F4. Neck Rolls—neck

F7. Arm Circles—arms and upper body

F11. The Lunge—groin and thighs

F12. Hurdles—groin and thighs

F15. Calf Stretches—lower legs

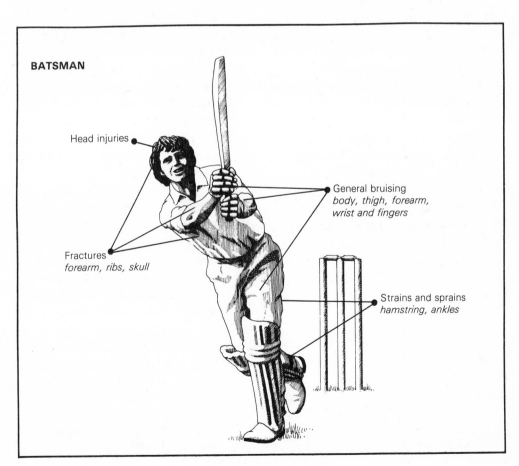

BATSMAN

Head injuries

General bruising
body, thigh, forearm, wrist and fingers

Fractures
forearm, ribs, skull

Strains and sprains
hamstring, ankles

In addition , **Clay (or Putty) Rolling** is a useful finger-flexing exercise. Take a piece of clay or putty the size of a squash ball (or a little smaller) and roll it around in the fingers, trying to make it as spherical as possible. Then flatten it and start again.

Strength
S1. Push-Ups or Modified Push-Ups—body
S2. Pull-Ups—arms and shoulders (*especially good for bowlers*)
S3. Two-Chair Push-Ups—arms and shoulders (*especially good for bowlers*)
S5. Broomstick Rolls—wrists and hands (*especially good for batsmen and bowlers*)
S6. Tennis Ball Squeeze—wrists and hands (*especially good for batsmen and bowlers*)
S10. Bent-Leg Sit-Ups—abdomen
S11. Half Squats—thighs (*especially good for bowlers and wicket keepers*)
S12. Squat Thrusts—thighs
S14. Paint Can Raises—upper legs (*especially good for wicket keepers*)
S17. Bench Jumps—upper legs

In addition, weight training under supervision, according to specific needs.

Heart and Lung
Running, particularly Fartlek, interval and sprint training, uphill or sandhill running. Intensive work should start about one month before the beginning of the season.
Jogging
Ropework

HOME CIRCUIT
Preliminary warm-up
Jogging on the spot
Ropework, if appropriate; otherwise jogging
F7. Arm Circles
S1. Push-Ups or Modified Push-Ups
F2. Trunk Twists
F11. The Lunge
S10. Bent-Leg Sit-Ups
S16. Step-Ups
F12. Hurdles
S17. Bench Jumps
S12. Squat Thrusts

CRICKET INJURIES
The most common cricket injuries are those caused by direct contact with the ball. This can cause considerable bruising, occasionally fractures.

General Bruising: Usually to the body, thigh, forearm, wrists and fingers for batsmen and wicket keepers. Wicket keepers often suffer from considerable hand bruising, and any cricketer may be hit on the foot by a ball and suffer bruising of the upper foot. Do not rule out fracture; if in any doubt have an X-ray.

Various forms of protective padding or shields, for thigh, forearm and so on, are on the market. Good batting gloves are essential. For wicket keepers an extra pair of inner gloves seems the only answer, but most look upon hand bruising as an occupational hazard.

Fractures (to Forearm, Ribs or Skull): These must be dealt with immediately by a doctor. A fieldsman's fingers can be broken if he fails to catch cleanly or if he falls.

Strains and Sprains: For fast bowlers (back) and wicket keepers (back and neck) these are occupational hazards. Pulled hamstrings or twisted ankles can result from sudden turning or twisting, but strength and flexibility exercises are a good safeguard. In some instances, bowling technique might place too great a strain on the back; if this is suspected get the advice of a cricket coach. To help prevent leg injuries make sure the boot studs are in good condition.

Bruised Heels: This is quite common in bowlers, especially fast bowlers, and is usually due to an incorrect placing of the lead foot when bowling. Orthotic foot devices could help.

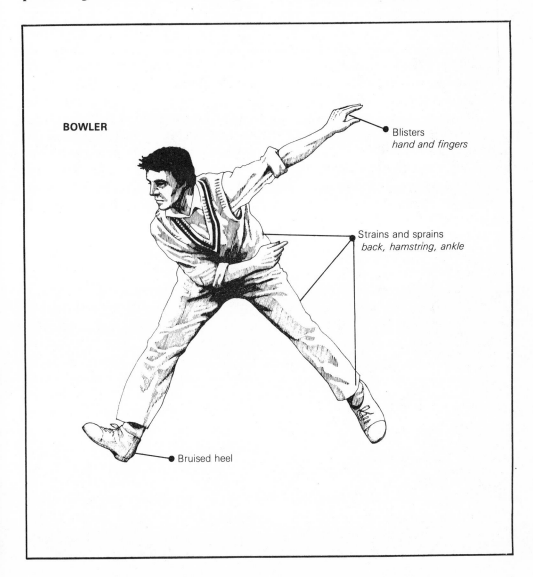

BOWLER

Blisters
hand and fingers

Strains and sprains
back, hamstring, ankle

Bruised heel

Basketball

BASKETBALL IS ONE OF THE most physically exacting sports, requiring stamina, speed, jumping ability, balance and timing. Considerable heart and lung endurance is needed to sustain the vigorous pace, and the explosive jumping power that is called for involves strength, especially in the trunk and legs. The start-stop nature of the game and the need for pivoting and the sudden dash requires both leg strength and flexibility in hips, knees and ankle joints. In addition, passing, dribbling and shooting calls for wrist and finger strength, as well as wrist flexibility.

Specifically, basketball demands a high standard of general fitness and stamina, allied to strength—especially in body, wrists and legs—and flexibility in the shoulders, wrists, fingers and legs.

Alternative Sports: The change-of-pace and start-stop nature of tennis, squash, badminton, volleyball and racquetball are all beneficial to the basketball player. Swimming and running are good for stamina building.

Warm-Up: The warm-up is extremely important in basketball. Off court this usually takes the form of jogging and gentle flexibility exercises, followed by on court passing, dribbling and shooting practice before the game.

BASKETBALL FITNESS EXERCISES

Flexibility
F2. Trunk Twists—trunk and neck
F4. Neck Rolls—neck
F7. Arm Circles—arms and shoulders
F9. Wrist Shakes—wrists and hands
F11. The Lunge—groin and thighs
F12. Hurdles—groin and thighs

Strength
S1. Push-Ups or Modified Push-Ups—body
S2. Pull-Ups—arms and shoulders
S5. Broomstick Rolls—wrists and hands
S8. Fingertip Hip Raises—fingers

S11. Half Squats—thighs
S12. Squat Thrusts—abdomen
S16. Step-Ups—upper legs
S19. Calf Raises—lower legs

In addition, **The Sitting Dribble** is a useful exercise. Sit in a chair and dribble a basketball on the floor on both sides and as far behind you as you can reach.

Heart and Lung
Running, especially Fartlek and interval training; sprints, zigzag and shuttle runs are also useful.
Jogging
Ropework

HOME CIRCUIT
Preliminary warm-up
Ropework, if appropriate; otherwise jogging

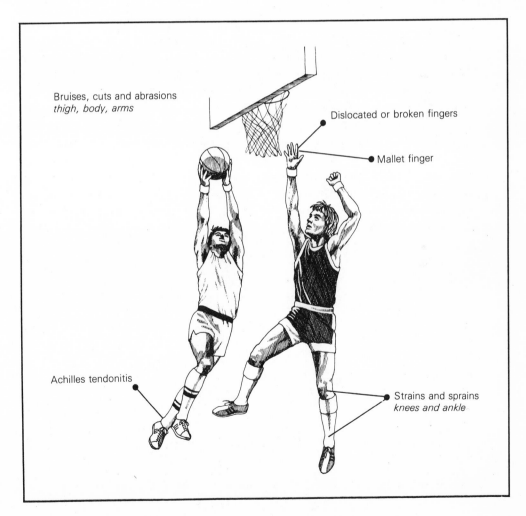

Bruises, cuts and abrasions
thigh, body, arms

Dislocated or broken fingers

Mallet finger

Achilles tendonitis

Strains and sprains
knees and ankle

S1. Push-Ups or Modified Push-Ups
F2. Trunk Twists
S11. Half Squats
S16. Step-Ups
F7. Arm Circles
F11. The Lunge
S12. Squat Thrusts

BASKETBALL INJURIES

Basketball injuries are quite common, as should be expected in a very fast game involving twisting and turning on an unyielding surface. Jumping places considerable strain on the legs, and the jarring effect of landing can lead to injuries of the feet and lower leg. Falling and collisions are another occupational risk of the game.

Bruises, Cuts and Abrasions: Particularly to the thigh, body and arms, largely due to falls. Some falls are outside the control of a player; others, however, are caused by slipping, so ensure that your shoes are in good repair with excellent soles.

Strains and Sprains: These are principally to the knee and ankle, and are usually caused by a too-sudden twist, turn or stop or by an awkward landing after a jump (the knee may also suffer cartilage trouble). Fingers may also suffer sprain or dislocation either in handling the ball, in falling or as a result of putting out a hand to save a fall. Flexibility and strength exercises in the conditioning program combined with a thorough warm-up before play should do much to avoid or minimize these injuries.

Mallet Finger: This may result when the ball strikes the end of the finger. The condition causes considerable pain and swelling; if the tendon holding the top joint is broken, the fingertip will droop. Treatment for mallet finger involves splinting for up to 6 weeks.

Achilles Tendonitis: This is a common injury in basketball. Flexibility exercises that focus on the lower leg will do much to prevent this from occurring. Inserting raised heels in the shoes may also help.

Netball

NETBALL IS A FAST-PACED game that requires considerable stamina as it consists of four 15-minute quarters with very little rest in between. Although at first sight it may appear similar to basketball, too close comparison is misleading as the court is less wide and rather longer and players must remain within their own areas. This calls for considerable passing skills as dribbling is not allowed.

Specifically, netball requires excellent heart and lung endurance; strength, especially in the legs (both for outjumping opponents and for the explosive speed and agility needed to cope with the start-stop and short-dash nature of play) as well as in arms, shoulder and neck; and flexibility in the hips (especially for pivoting), shoulders, arms, wrists, fingers and legs.

Alternative Sports: Tennis, squash and badminton are all popular alternative or off-season sports as they help maintain general fitness and improve the essential hand/eye and start-stop coordination needed in netball. For learning how to fall correctly on a hard surface, judo, aikido and (for men) wrestling are useful.

Warm-Up: Extensive warming-up is essential in a sport in which the player is plunged into explosive activity from the outset. **Off court**, carry out flexibility exercises with emphasis on trunk, shoulders and legs. **On court**, practice should include some jogging around the court, ending with sprints down the total length of one side during the last laps and then netball skills, such as throwing, catching and changing speed and direction.

NETBALL FITNESS EXERCISES
Flexibility
F1. Side Bends—hips and thighs
F2. Trunk Twists—trunk and neck
F4. Neck Rolls—neck
F5. Shoulder Shrugs—shoulders
F7. Arm Circles—arms and upper body
F9. Wrist Shakes—wrist
F11. The Lunge—groin and thighs

Strength

S1. Push-Ups or Modified Push-Ups
—body

S5. Broomstick Rolls—wrists and hands

S10. Bent-Leg Sit-Ups—abdomen

S12. Squat Thrusts—thighs

S16. Step-Ups—upper legs

S17. Bench Jumps—upper legs

S19. Calf Raises—lower legs

In addition, weight training under supervision: low-resistance, high-repetition exercises with emphasis on shoulder, neck, arms and legs.

Heart and Lung

Running, including Fartlek and interval training, shuttle runs, zigzags and windsprints

Jogging

Ropework

HOME CIRCUIT

Preliminary warm-up

Ropework, if appropriate; otherwise jogging

F2. Trunk Twists

S1. Push-Ups or Modified Push-Ups

F11. The Lunge

S19. Calf Raises

F7. Arm Circles

S16. Step-Ups

S10. Bent-Leg Sit-Ups

F5. Shoulder Shrugs

NETBALL INJURIES

Abrasions: Especially to hands, forearms and thighs, these are often due to falls.

Blisters (Feet): These are particularly prevalent at the start of the season. It is important to harden the feet before starting to play in earnest.

Strains and Sprains: The knee and ankle are especially vulnerable. Sprains and strains occur either in falls, or as a result of a sudden turn or twist. Occasionally they are the result of landing awkwardly or on another player's foot. Flexibility and strength exercises in the conditioning program and a really thorough warm-up should do much to lessen the likelihood of such injuries.

Fingers and Wrists: Sprains, occasionally fractures. These are usually due to a fall or an attempt to prevent a fall. Knee-, ankle- and wrist-strengthening exercises do a lot to prevent these injuries.

Mallet Finger: This is caused by failing to catch a ball cleanly. The ball strikes the end of the finger and, in addition to causing considerable pain and swelling, may break the tendon affixed to the top joint, causing the fingertip to droop. Treatment involves splinting for up to 6 weeks.

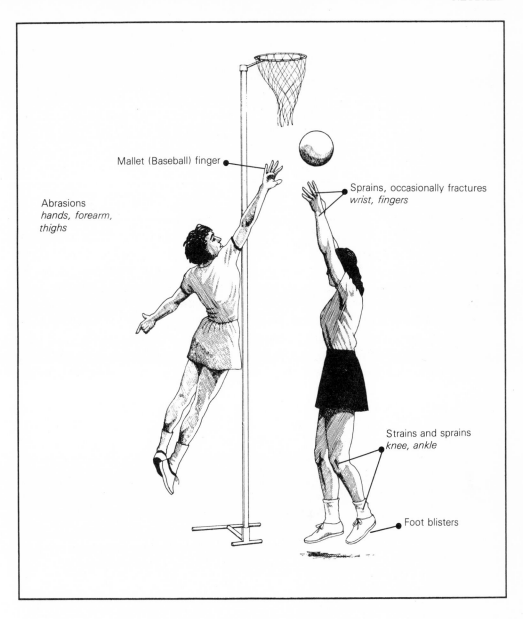

Mallet (Baseball) finger

Abrasions
hands, forearm, thighs

Sprains, occasionally fractures
wrist, fingers

Strains and sprains
knee, ankle

Foot blisters

Football

FOOTBALL IS A HIGHLY PHYSICAL sport requiring a good standard of general fitness. It involves constant body contact, with opposing players running at each other at high speed. To avoid injury, football players need to be in top shape. Although running stamina is very important in a game of such long duration, the primary running requirement is an ability to perform many short sprints involving explosive bursts of speed.

Specific fitness for football demands good heart and lung endurance; strength, particularly in the neck, trunk, shoulders and legs (especially thighs, knees and ankles); and flexibility in the back and chest, shoulders and legs.

Alternative Sports: Running, swimming, cycling and jogging are all useful stamina builders. Racquet sports, such as tennis, badminton and squash, as well as basketball, handball and golf are good general conditioners.

Warm-Up: This should include jogging and running in place, followed by flexibility exercises until a good sweat has been built up. To keep limber on the sidelines, running on the spot every 5 minutes is useful. It is important to remain warmly dressed until actually called on to the field.

FOOTBALL FITNESS
EXERCISES
Flexibility

F1. Side Bends—hips and thighs
F2. Trunk Twists—trunk and neck
F3. Alternate Toe Touches—back, shoulders and arms
F4. Neck Rolls—neck
F6. Wing Stretchers—shoulders

F8. Arm Flings—arms and upper body
F11. The Lunge—groin and thigh
F12. Hurdles—groin and thigh
F14. Knee Pulls—lower leg

Strength

S1. Push Ups—body
S2. Pull-Ups—arms and shoulders
S3. Two-Chair Push-Ups—arms and shoulders
S6. Tennis Ball Squeeze—wrists and hands
S7. Fingertip Push-Ups—fingers
S11. Half Squats—thighs
S15. Leg Raises—upper leg
S16. Step-Ups—upper leg
S17. Bench Jumps—upper leg
S19. Calf Raises—lower leg

In addition, weight training under supervision, especially for neck, shoulders, back and legs: high-resistance, low-repetition in the off-season period; low-resistance, high-repetition during the season.

Heart and Lung

Running, especially Fartlek and interval training; sprints (from 15 yards, increasing up to 40 yards); zigzag running; shuttle runs; running uphill; running up stadium steps
Swimming
Ropework

HOME CIRCUIT

Running in place
Ropework, if appropriate, otherwise jogging
S1. Push-Ups
F2. Trunk Twists
S11. Half Squats
S16. Step-Ups
F3. Alternate Toe Touches
F11. The Lunge
S7. Fingertip Push-Ups
S16. Step-Ups

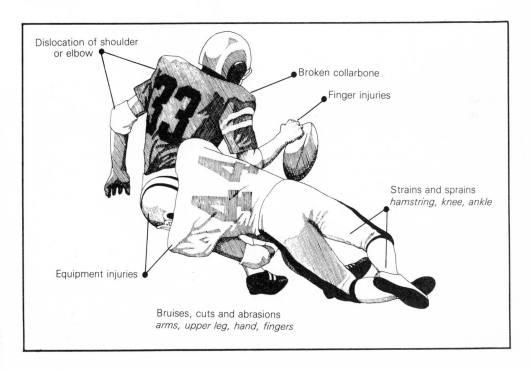

Dislocation of shoulder or elbow

Broken collarbone

Finger injuries

Strains and sprains
hamstring, knee, ankle

Equipment injuries

Bruises, cuts and abrasions
arms, upper leg, hand, fingers

FOOTBALL INJURIES

Bruises, cuts and abrasions are common football injuries. Most vulnerable are the arms and upper legs, as well as the hands and fingers. Linemen often tape fingers and knuckles as a preventative to superficial hand injuries. The fingers are also vulnerable to more severe injuries, either in failing to catch the ball cleanly or from contact with another player.

Falling injuries can also cause damage to the wrist or fingers, as well as dislocation of the elbow or shoulder or a broken collarbone. It is essential to learn how to fall properly, which is why a good number of football players also take up judo, aikido or wrestling.

Strains and sprains are quite common in football. Particularly vulnerable are the ankles, knees and hamstrings. Quick twists and turns are usually responsible; sometimes rough or slippery ground can also cause such injuries. Taping of the ankle is a good preventative. To help prevent hamstring pulls, it is essential to carry out balanced exercises for the quadriceps muscles at the front of the thigh and the hamstrings at the back.

In general, many strains and sprains can be prevented or at least minimized by ensuring that the general conditioning includes a full range of flexibility and strength exercises for parts of the body most at risk, combined with thorough warm-up before play.

Protective clothing injuries are commonly caused by the helmet (as in spearing) or by the shoulder pads and can lead to internal injuries or wrenched muscles. In addition, ill-fitting or defective equipment is also responsible for many football injuries. It is essential that protective gear be kept in top condition.

Soccer

SOCCER CAN BE ENJOYED at all levels of expertise. It carries less premium on size and strength than many other sports and requires no elaborate preparation. Increasingly, it has come to be looked upon as an excellent alternative sport by many athletes, as it develops all-around athletic ability, builds stamina and improves body coordination, footwork, agility and ball control, all with considerably less risk of injury than in many other sports—especially when the game is played for exercise, with rubber-soled (as opposed to studded) shoes.

Enjoying soccer to the fullest requires a reasonable degree of prior fitness, as the game consists of 90 minutes of almost continuous action, with a single break of only 5 minutes.

Specifically, soccer demands a high degree of heart and lung endurance; strength in the whole body, but especially in the upper trunk and legs (because running power is all-important); and flexibility in the lower body and in the upper and lower legs, particularly in the hamstrings and calves.

Alternative Sports: Running, jogging and cycling are all useful stamina builders. Basketball, rugby and team handball are good for developing speed, stamina and agility as well as for teaching positional play. Squash is the best all-around exercise.

Warm-Up: Jogging, followed by flexibility exercises off the field. This should be succeeded by windsprints and soccer-skill drills (kicking, heading, passing, etc.) carried out on a surface similar to the one you are about to play on.

These exercises should be performed wearing boots that are only loosely laced. Tighten them after the warm-up.

SOCCER FITNESS EXERCISES
Flexibility
F1. Side Bends—hips and thighs
F2. Trunk Twists—trunk and neck
F3. Alternate Toe Touches—back, shoulders and arms
F7. Arm Circles—arms and upper body
F11. The Lunge—groin and thigh
F12. Hurdles—groin and thigh
F14. Knee Pulls—lower leg

Strength
S1. Push-Ups or Modified Push-Ups —body
S2. Pull-Ups—arms and shoulders
S9. "Bicycling"—abdomen

S10. Bent-Leg Sit-Ups—abdomen
S12. Squat Thrusts—thighs
S15. Leg Raises—upper legs
S16. Step-Ups—upper legs
S18. Shin Strengtheners—lower legs

In addition, weight training under supervision, especially for body and legs.

Heart and Lung
Running, including Fartlek and interval training; sprints up to 25 yards and shuttle runs up to 150 yards
Cycling
Jogging
Ropework

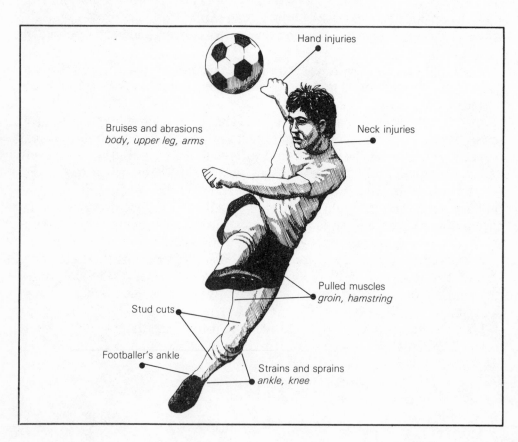

Hand injuries

Neck injuries

Bruises and abrasions
body, upper leg, arms

Pulled muscles
groin, hamstring

Stud cuts

Footballer's ankle

Strains and sprains
ankle, knee

HOME CIRCUIT
Preliminary warm-up
Ropework, if appropriate; otherwise
  jogging
F2. Trunk Twists
S1. Push-Ups or Modified Push-Ups
F7. Arm Circles
S9. "Bicycling"
S2. Pull-Ups
F11. The Lunge
S10. Bent-Leg Sit-Ups
F14. Knee Pulls
S12. Squat Thrusts

SOCCER INJURIES
These are most commonly to the legs and ankles; and are usually caused by sudden twists or turns, uneven ground, miskicks or the action of another player.

Bruises and abrasions: especially to the body, upper leg and arm. Cuts and abrasions can easily become infected unless dealt with competently. In addition, **burns** can occur in falling on some of the artificial surfaces that are coming increasingly into use.

Hand Injuries: These occur in falling, or when a player puts out a hand to prevent a fall, which can also lead to dislocated shoulders or even a broken collarbone, especially on hard ground. Goalkeepers frequently suffer hand sprains or foot fractures while catching or otherwise stopping the ball, or as a result of colliding with their own goalposts.

Strains and Sprains: Ankle and knee sprains are due either to a sudden twist, turn or stop, a miskick or an attempt to kick a blocked ball. Sometimes these can lead to a displaced cartilage in the knee, or a strained (even ruptured) Achilles tendon.

Hamstring or groin pulls: These are usually due to overstretching while trying to reach a ball. Hamstring injuries are made more likely by overstrengthening the quadriceps muscles at the front of the thigh at the expense of the hamstrings at the back. Balanced flexibility and strength exercises will do much to minimize these and other strain injuries.

Footballer's Ankle: This is a highly troublesome condition that is due to constantly kicking the ball when the foot is flexed downward. Foot-strengthening and flexibility exercises are a good preventive measure, as is getting the advice of a coach on kicking technique.

Stud Cuts: These are usually confined to the lower leg and thigh, especially to the calves. They may be quite deep and can also easily become infected, so like all cuts on the soccer field they must be dealt with quickly and competently.

Neck Injuries: These are sometimes caused by bad heading of the ball, and they can be serious. Any suspicion of a sore neck due to poor heading should be seen to by a doctor without delay. Training and experience make the chances of such injuries less likely.

Rugby

RUGBY IS A FAST CONTACT GAME requiring a high degree of general fitness, body coordination and ball control. In training for a fast, almost nonstop game of 80 minutes with only a 5-minute break, great emphasis must be placed on developing a player's stamina to combat the fatigue which in turn can lead to injury. The rugby player must also be ready for short bursts of intense activity lasting on average from 10–20 seconds.

Specific fitness for rugby involves a high level of heart and lung endurance; strength, especially in the body and legs (for tackling and resisting tackles, as well as for providing the necessary side-stepping and accelerating ability): and flexibility in the trunk, arms and lower limbs.

Physical fitness requirements vary with position. **Tight forwards** need strength, especially in the legs, back and arms for scrummages, rucks and mauls. **Back row forwards** must be speedy and strong, especially in the arms and shoulders. **Backs** must be fast and capable of explosive bursts of speed. This calls for strength, especially in the shoulders and legs.

Alternative Sports: Running, jogging, swimming and cycling are all good for stamina building. Squash, tennis, badminton, basketball and volleyball are useful for improving agility, acceleration and ball control.

Warm-Up: This usually consists of some jogging, jogging on the spot and some sprinting practice, followed by flexibility exercises, passing practices and other rugby skill drills.

RUGBY FITNESS EXERCISES
Flexibility

F1. Side Bends—hips and thighs
F2. Trunk Twists—trunk and neck
F3. Alternate Toe Touches—back, shoulders and arms
F4. Neck Rolls—neck
F7. Arm Circles—arms and upper trunk
F12. Hurdles—groin and thighs
F14. Knee Pulls—lower leg
F15. Calf Stretches—lower leg

Strength

S1. Push-Ups—body

S2. Pull-Ups—arms and shoulders

S3. Two-Chair Push-Ups—arms and shoulders

S5. Broomstick Rolls—hands and wrists

S10. Bent-Leg Sit-Ups—abdomen

S12. Squat Thrusts—thighs

S16. Step-Ups—upper leg

S17. Bench Jumps—upper leg

In addition, weight training under supervision, especially for the trunk and legs.

Heart and Lung

Running—especially Fartlek and interval training; sprints and shuttle runs are good for developing speed, acceleration and agility

Jogging   Swimming

Ropework   Cycling

HOME CIRCUIT

Preliminary Warm-Up

Jogging on the spot

Ropework, if appropriate; otherwise jogging

S1. Push-Ups

F2. Trunk Twists

F12. Hurdles

S16. Step-Ups

F4. Neck Rolls

S12. Squat Thrusts

F3. Alternate Toe Touches

S10. Bent-Leg Sit-Ups

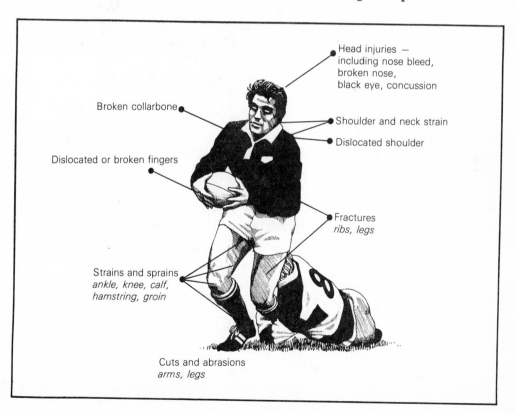

Head injuries — including nose bleed, broken nose, black eye, concussion

Broken collarbone

Shoulder and neck strain

Dislocated shoulder

Dislocated or broken fingers

Fractures
ribs, legs

Strains and sprains
ankle, knee, calf, hamstring, groin

Cuts and abrasions
arms, legs

RUGBY INJURIES

In such a vigorous contact game as rugby, in which play is often on rough or slippery surfaces and violence can occur unless there is strict and vigilant refereeing, injuries are frequent. More particularly, however, to forwards rather than backs.

Many parts of the body are vulnerable. **Bruises, cuts and abrasions** are common especially to the arms and legs. These can easily become infected unless dealt with competently.

Strains and sprains are frequent, particularly at the start of the season. The ankles and knees are most vulnerable, although the calf, groin and hamstring are also often affected. Hamstring pulls often occur in overreaching when picking up the ball, or if the foot slips.

In the scrummage, shoulder and neck sprains can also occur. The wrist can also be sprained (occasionally fractured) in falls or when a player tries to save himself from a fall. (On hard ground this can also lead to a broken collarbone.)

Most strains and sprains, if not avoided altogether, can certainly be minimized by a proper conditioning program including a full range of stretching and strengthening exercises for the most vulnerable parts of the body, combined with a really thorough warm-up before play.

Hard tackling can account for **ankle and knee injuries** and occasionally **shoulder dislocations**. **Fingers** are often **dislocated or broken** while handling the ball or through kicks on the hand during play. **Fractures** can also be sustained, particularly to the legs and ribs.

Head injuries are also quite frequent. These can range from nose bleeds, broken noses, cut lips and black eyes to concussion.

Field Hockey

FIELD HOCKEY IS A GAME requiring power, speed and good body coordination. It is conducted at a very fast pace, and the hockey player is called upon for sudden bursts of speed and frequent changes of direction and start-stop movements.

Specifically, the hockey player requires considerable heart and lung endurance; strength, particularly in the lower body and legs; and flexibility in the hips, lower limbs and wrists. Goalkeepers require greater physical strength than forwards or backs, as well as lighting quick reactions.

Alternative Sports: Squash, tennis, soccer and golf are all popular off-season or alternative sports among hockey players. As many injuries are caused in falling, learning how to fall without injury is important to hockey players. Accordingly, some take up judo, aikido or wrestling.

Warm-Up: The hockey warm-up usually takes the form of gentle jogging and flexibility exercises off the field, followed by passing, shooting and other hockey-skill drills. A high level of general body suppleness combined with thorough warming-up before a match has startling effects in reducing hockey injuries.

HOCKEY FITNESS EXERCISES

Flexibility
F1. Side Bends—hips and thighs
F2. Trunk Twists—trunk and neck
F4. Neck Rolls—neck
F7. Arm Circles—arms and upper trunk
F11. The Lunge—groin and thighs
F12. Hurdles—groin and thighs
F15. Calf Stretches—lower legs

Strength
S1. Push-Ups or Modified Push-Ups —body
S2. Pull-Ups—arms and shoulders
S5. Broomstick Rolls—wrists and hands
S10. Bent-Leg Sit-Ups—abdomen
S11. Half Squats—thighs
S17. Bench Jumps—upper legs

In addition, weight training under supervision, especially for the lower trunk and legs.

Heart and Lung
Running, particularly Fartlek and interval training; and shuttle runs and sprints (for improving speed)
Jogging
Ropework

HOME CIRCUIT
Preliminary warm-up
Jogging on the spot
Ropework, if appropriate, otherwise jogging

F2. Trunk Twists
S1. Push-Ups or Modified Push-Ups
F11. The Lunge
S2. Pull-Ups
F1 Side Bends
F7. Arm Circles
S10. Bent-Leg Sit-Ups
S17. Bench Jumps

HOCKEY INJURIES
Bruises: Particularly on the thigh, forearms, wrists, hands and fingers are quite common in hockey and are usually caused by contact with stick or ball, occasionally due to collision with another player.

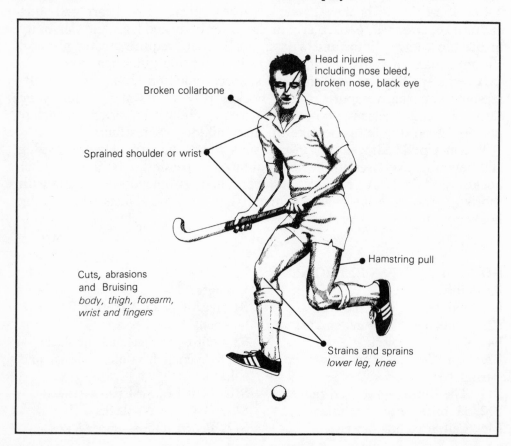

Head injuries — including nose bleed, broken nose, black eye

Broken collarbone

Sprained shoulder or wrist

Hamstring pull

Cuts, abrasions and Bruising
body, thigh, forearm, wrist and fingers

Strains and sprains
lower leg, knee

Cuts and Abrasions: These also occur frequently, as do**burns,** caused by falling on some of the newer artificial surfaces, which are becoming increasingly common.

Wrist and Shoulder Sprains, Broken Collarbones: These are frequently the result of falling, especially on hard ground.

Strains and Sprains (particularly to the lower leg and knee) **and Hamstring Pulls:** These occur as a result of a slip or overstretching to reach a ball. Hamstring pulls are often made more likely by imbalance between the relative muscle strengths of the quadriceps muscles at the front of the thigh and the hamstrings at the back. This can be remedied by a program of balanced strength and flexibility exercises for the two muscle groups. Proper conditioning and a really thorough warm-up should lessen the chance of injury.

Head Injuries: These vary from nose bleed, occasional broken noses and black eyes. They are often due to the ball flying up during a clash of sticks or after it hits rough ground.

Lacrosse

LACROSSE IS ONE OF the fastest team games in the world. It calls for a high standard of general fitness, speed of an explosive and start-stop nature, and the ability to twist, turn and pivot often at high speed and in full stride. Women's lacrosse differs from men's International Lacrosse in that it does not allow contact between players; it is therefore a more flowing, rhythmic game, but there is little difference in the physical requirements.

Specific fitness for lacrosse involves considerable heart and lung endurance; strength, especially in the back, arms, wrists and legs; and flexibility in the body, arms, wrists and legs.

Alternative Sports: Racquet sports, particularly squash and badminton, and basketball are all excellent for helping hand/eye coordination and ball control. Swimming, running, jogging and other team sports such as soccer and handball are good for stamina building.

Warm-Up: This should take the form of some gentle jogging, followed by stretching exercises off the field. On the field, catching, throwing and goal-shooting exercises should precede the game.

LACROSSE FITNESS
EXERCISES
Flexibility

F1. Side Bends—hips and thighs
F2. Trunk Twists—trunk and neck
F4. Neck Rolls—neck
F5. Shoulder Shrugs—shoulders
F7. Arm Circles—arms and upper trunk
F9. Wrist Shakes—wrists and hands
F11. The Lunge—groin and thighs
F12. Hurdles—groin and thighs

In addition, a popular lacrosse flexibility exercise is **Stick Twists.** Hold the lacrosse stick above the head, with the hands 2 feet apart. Bring it down behind the head and then carry out twisting movements from side to side and up and down.

Strength

S1. Push-Ups or Modified Push-Ups
—body

S5. Broomstick Rolls—wrists and
hands

S10. Bent-Leg Sit-Ups—abdomen

S11. Half Squats—thighs

S13. Sprinters—thighs

S14. Paint-Can Raises—upper leg

S19. Calf Raises—lower leg

In addition, weight training under supervision

Heart and Lung

Running, including Fartlek and interval training, sprint training and shuttle runs

Swimming   Ropework

HOME CIRCUIT

Preliminary warm-up

Jogging on the spot

Ropework, if appropriate; otherwise jogging

F2. Trunk Twists

S1. Push-Ups or Modified Push-Ups

F11. The Lunge

S14. Paint-Can Raises

F7. Arm Circles

S10. Bent-Leg Sit-Ups

F1. Side Bends

S13. Sprinters

LACROSSE INJURIES

The extensive padding and protective gear (especially the helmet with faceguard) worn in men's lacrosse pre-

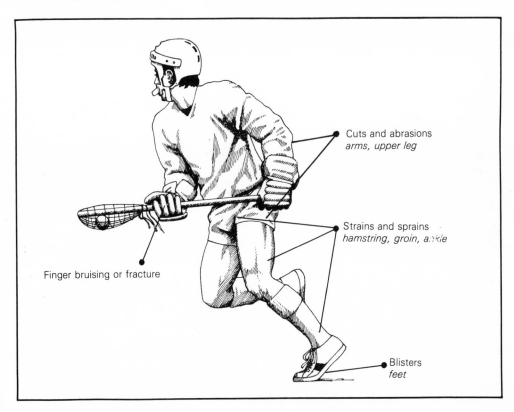

Cuts and abrasions
arms, upper leg

Strains and sprains
hamstring, groin, ankle

Finger bruising or fracture

Blisters
feet

vents many injuries. Despite this, lacrosse players are still frequently subject to injuries, especially those that result from blows by a stick or ball.

Bruising can be quite severe, especially to the thighs and legs. Despite the gloves that are worn (in men's lacrosse only, except for goalies in women's lacrosse), bruises to the hands and occasionally **finger fractures** also occur. Women players are often hit severely on the knuckles by opponents' sticks, and, though more rarely, by the ball.

Cuts and abrasions due to falls are quite common. And, as with many types of new surface, **burns** can also occur, the arms and upper legs being most vulnerable.

Blisters on the feet are particularly prevalent in hot weather or at the start of the season before feet have become adequately hardened.

Strains and sprains, particularly of the hamstring, groin or ankle, are quite common injuries. These can be largely avoided with proper conditioning and a really thorough warm-up before a game.

Team Handball

TEAM HANDBALL IS ONE OF the world's fastest team games, requiring great speed, agility, body coordination and ball control.

Specific fitness for team handball requires a high level of heart and lung endurance; strength, particularly in the legs and thighs, upper arms and wrists; and flexibility in the legs, arms and wrists, as well as in the lower trunk for the jumping, pivoting and diving that the game calls for.

Alternative Sports: Running, jogging, swimming and ropework are excellent stamina builders. Some players prefer team games; soccer is especially popular. Basketball requires very similar skills and footwork, and volleyball is also useful. Gymnastics is perhaps the best alternative or off-season sport to provide the body suppleness the team handball player requires.

Warm-Up: In such an instantly explosive sport as handball, the warm-up is of crucial importance. This usually consists of some gentle jogging followed by flexibility exercises, all conducted off court. On-court warm-up is usually more extensive and the whole warm-up routine can last for 30–45 minutes. On-court warm-up includes passing, catching, goal shooting and general ball-control drills.

TEAM HANDBALL FITNESS EXERCISES

Flexibility

F2. Trunk Twists—trunk and neck

F3. Alternate Toe Touches—back, shoulders and arms

F4. Neck Rolls—neck

F7. Arm Circles—arms and upper trunk

F9. Wrist Shakes—wrists and hands

F11. The Lunge—groin and thighs

F12. Hurdles—groin and thighs

F14. Knee Pulls—lower legs

Strength

S1. Push-Ups or Modified Push-Ups
   —body
S5. Broomstick Rolls—wrists and
   hands
S6. Tennis Ball Squeeze—wrists and
   hands
S8. Fingertip Hip Raises—fingers
S10. Bent-Leg Sit-Ups—abdomen
S16. Step-Ups—upper leg
S17. Bench Jumps—upper leg
S19. Calf Raises—lower leg

In addition, weight training under supervision, with emphasis on legs, thighs, upper arms and wrists.

Heart and Lung

Running, especially Fartlek and interval training, shuttle runs and sprint training
Jogging
Swimming
Ropework

HOME CIRCUIT

Preliminary warm-up
Jogging on the spot
Ropework if appropriate; otherwise jogging
S1. Push-Ups or Modified Push-Ups
S10. Bent-Leg Sit-Ups
F4. Neck Rolls

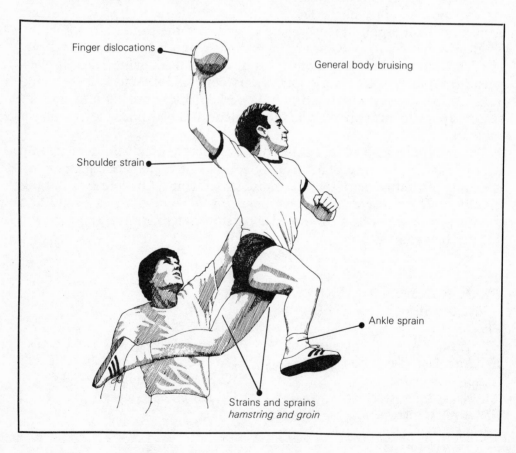

Finger dislocations

General body bruising

Shoulder strain

Ankle sprain

Strains and sprains
hamstring and groin

F11. The Lunge
F2. Trunk Twists
S16. Step-Ups
F7. Arm Circles
S17. Bench Jumps

TEAM HANDBALL INJURIES
General body bruising may arise from falls or slips or occasional body contact. Twists, turns and sudden pivoting can lead to **hamstring and groin strains**, sometimes a **twisted ankle**. Throwing the ball or punching it can result in **shoulder strain**; as with other strains and sprains, all of these can largely be avoided by proper conditioning and a really thorough warm-up before play.

The **fingers** may also be either **dislocated or wrenched** either in falls, or preventing a fall, or as a result of not catching the ball cleanly.

In addition, on some artificial surfaces players are suffering from **burns** as a result of falls. To prevent this, practice games should be carried out wearing trousers and long-sleeved shirts. It is also of value for players to learn to fall properly. For this judo, aikido or wrestling are useful alternative sports.

Court Handball

COURT HANDBALL IS AN IMMENSELY fast game requiring a high degree of general fitness. It is particularly popular for those who find racquet sports difficult but want a quick, intensive workout. The physical agility demanded is very high, and the frequent stooping and reaching calls for considerable body suppleness combined with nimble footwork and excellent body coordination.

Specific fitness for court handball involves a high degree of heart and lung endurance; strength, particularly in the lower trunk, legs, arms and wrists; and flexibility in the trunk and shoulders, arms and wrists.

Alternative Sports: Running, jogging and swimming are all good stamina builders; best of all is ropework, which is also excellent for improving general agility. Basketball and volleyball promote suppleness, and aikido and judo are invaluable aids to speeding the reactions and reflexes.

Warm-Up: In such an intensely energetic game as court handball, the warm-up is very important indeed. Most players carry out some light jogging followed by flexibility exercises, especially for the lower back, arms and wrists. On-court warm-up should include a general work-up to the amount of exertion likely to be involved in the game.

COURT HANDBALL FITNESS EXERCISES

Flexibility
F1. Side Bends—hips and thighs
F2. Trunk Twists—trunk and neck
F3. Alternate Toe Touches—back, shoulders and arms
F4. Neck Rolls—neck
F9. Wrist Shakes—wrists and hands
F11. The Lunge—groin and thighs

F14. Knee Pulls—lower legs
F15. Calf Stretches—lower legs

Strength
S1. Push-Ups or Modified Push-Ups —body
S2. Pull-Ups—arms and shoulders

S5. Broomstick Rolls—wrists and hands

S6. Tennis Ball Squeeze—wrists and hands

S10. Bent-Leg Sit-Ups—abdomen

S16. Step-Ups—upper leg

S17. Bench Jumps—upper leg

S19. Calf Raises—lower leg

In addition, weight training under supervision, especially for lower trunk, legs, arms and wrists.

Heart and Lung

Running, particularly Fartlek and interval training, shuttle runs and zigzags

Jogging

Swimming

Ropework

HOME CIRCUIT

Preliminary warm-up

Jogging in place

Ropework, if appropriate; otherwise jogging

S1. Push-Ups or Modified Push-Ups

F2. Trunk Twists

F11. The Lunge

S2. Pull-Ups

F14. Knee Pulls

S10. Bent-Leg Sit-Ups

F3. Alternate Toe Touches

S17. Bench Jumps

COURT HANDBALL INJURIES

Hand Bruising: This is probably the most prevalent injury in court handball. Some players tape or bandage their hands before play, others prefer to

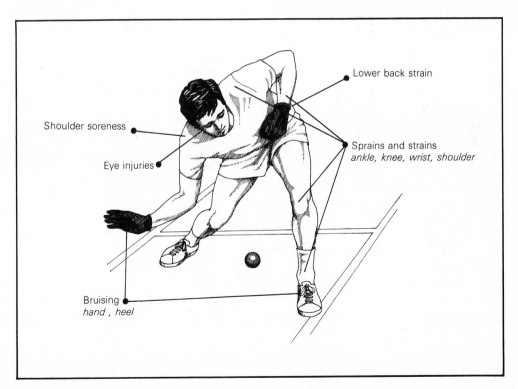

Shoulder soreness

Eye injuries

Bruising
hand , heel

Lower back strain

Sprains and strains
ankle, knee, wrist, shoulder

rely on thick inner gloves. Confidence and experience will diminish the incidence of this injury, but it still occurs with even the best players.

Sprains and Strains: The ankle and knee are particularly susceptible due to the speed and start-stop nature of the game. Also vulnerable are the wrist and the shoulder, which can be dislocated. Intensive flexibility and strengthening exercises as well as a thorough warm-up before play should do much to avoid or minimize these injuries.

Lower Back Strain: This is caused by the constant stooping and reaching that the game demands. Conditioning should include flexibility and strengthening exercises for the back.

Bruised Heels: These are quite common in court handball. Padded heel cups should ease the discomfort and lessen the chance of recurrence.

Shoulder Soreness: This is usually eased by taking a hot bath or shower and gently kneading the muscles and joint under water. This should eliminate most of the discomfort and prevent stiffness the next day.

Eye Injuries: These can be very severe in court handball. There is a strong case for wearing eye protectors or guards during play.

Volleyball

VOLLEYBALL IS A GAME that calls for a very high standard of general fitness. Conducted at a fast pace, it requires frequent short explosive bursts of speed and the ability to jump high and smash hard, which demands a high degree of agility and all-round suppleness. Much of the game is played in a moving half- or three-quarter-stoop position, which places exhausting demands on the body. Spiking in particular, places a great strain on the abdomen.

Specific fitness for volleyball involves considerable heart and lung endurance; strength in the back, shoulders, arms, wrists and legs, particularly in the jumping muscles (the quadriceps and hamstrings); and flexibility in the body generally and in the legs and arms.

Alternative Sports: Handball and basketball are the two favorite alternative or off-season sports for the volleyball player. Swimming is a good exercise for arm strengthening, racquet sports, however, tend to make the arms too stiff. Judo, aikido and wrestling are useful in helping to teach the player how to fall without injury. Certain athletic field events, such as the long and triple jump, call for muscle action similar to that in the spiking movement, and as such are useful vehicles for developing spiking skill.

Warm-Up: The warm-up is essential in such an immediately explosive game as volleyball. This usually takes the form of off-court jogging and flexibility exercises, followed by on-court practice particularly in passing and spiking.

VOLLEYBALL FITNESS EXERCISES

Flexibility
F1. Side Bends—hips and thighs
F2. Trunk Twists—trunk and neck
F4. Neck Rolls—neck
F7. Arm Circles—arms and upper body
F9. Wrist Shakes—wrists and hands
F12. Hurdles—groin and thighs

Strength

S1. Push-Ups or Modified Push-Ups —body

S2. Pull-Ups—arms and shoulders

S5. Broomstick Rolls—wrists and hands

S6. Tennis Ball Squeeze—wrists and hands

S8. Fingertip Hip Raises—fingers

S10. Bent-Leg Sit-Ups—abdomen

S11. Half Squats—thighs

S17. Bench Jumps—upper legs

In addition, weight training under supervision, with emphasis on back, shoulders, arms and wrists, and particularly the upper leg.

Heart and Lung

Running, particularly Fartlek, interval and sprint training (10–15 yards optimum)

Jogging

Ropework

In addition, volleyball players practice diving forwards on to the hands and also shoulder-roll falling.

HOME CIRCUIT

Preliminary warm-up

Jogging on the spot

Ropework, if appropriate; otherwise jogging

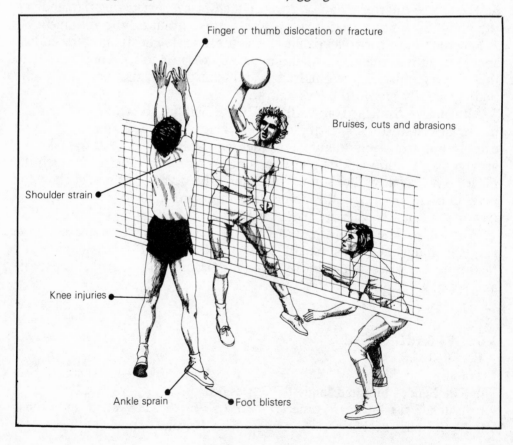

Finger or thumb dislocation or fracture

Bruises, cuts and abrasions

Shoulder strain

Knee injuries

Ankle sprain

Foot blisters

S1. Push-Ups or Modified Push-Ups
F2. Trunk Twists
S2. Pull-Ups
F12. Hurdles
S17. Bench Jumps
S10. Bent-Leg Sit-Ups
F7. Arm Circles
S11. Half Squats

VOLLEYBALL INJURIES

Bruises, Cuts and Abrasions: These are probably the most frequent volleyball injuries and are usually the result of falls. Some artificial surfaces are also inclined to give bad **burns**.

Blisters to the Foot: These are apt to be troublesome at the start of the season, and it is well worth while setting about hardening the feet in good time. Extra padding inside the shoe may also help.

Sprains: These occur to the shoulder during spiking and to the ankle as a result of a sudden twist, turn or awkward landing (as on another player's foot). They can largely be prevented by proper conditioning and a thorough warm-up before a game. **Knee injuries**, especially wrenched knees or displaced cartilages, are also known.

Fractures: These are not frequent, but when they occur they are usually to the fingers or the thumb, which may also suffer dislocation. They are either the result of a fall or awkard contact with the ball on the outstretched hand.

Golf

GOLF, DESPITE BEING one of the most popular amateur sporting activities is, from the fitness angle, almost totally neglected. Most casual players make for the course as soon as they can, hurry to the tee to forestall a long wait and, after only the most perfunctory of practice swings, blast off hoping to drive the ball into the next county. Some may do so without injury, but many do not, and few golfers appreciate the importance of golf fitness not only in injury prevention, but in improving their game and their enjoyment of it.

Golf is a very physical sport. It requires considerable heart and lung endurance to withstand general fatigue and enable a golfer to maintain rhythm and alertness over a long eighteen holes on a very hot day if a golf cart isn't being used—and many players now prefer to walk. Strength is needed, especially in the back, shoulders, forearms, wrists and fingers. Flexibility is required in the hips, shoulders and wrists, and lower legs.

Alternative Sports: Jogging, running, swimming and cycling are all excellent for stamina building. Racquet sports (though some coaches consider it a mistake to play one-armed games over prolonged periods), volleyball, handball and basketball all aid general fitness and keep the golfing muscles in trim.

Warm-Up: To drive off with full power at the start of the day—especially if the weather is cold—is to ask for muscle aches and pains and more serious injuries. Warming-up should include a little jogging followed by stretching exercises, especially for the back and legs. This should be succeeded by some two-club swinging (both clubs in the same hand) and then a 10-minute practice, starting off with a short club (a 7 or 8 iron), to establish rhythm and loosen tight muscles.

GOLF EXERCISES
Flexibility
F1. Side Bends—hips and thighs
F2. Trunk Twists—trunk and neck
F3. Alternate Toe Touches—back, shoulders and arms
F7. Arm Circles—arms and upper body
F9. Wrist Shakes—wrists
F11. The Lunge—groin and thigh
F13. Leg Swings—upper leg
F14. Knee Pulls—lower leg

In addition, try this variation of Trunk Twists (F2): place a golf club across the shoulders and behind the neck and carry out trunk twisting in that position.

Try also **Body Swings**. Place a golf club across the small of the back and lock it with both elbows. Then practice your swing as though you had a club in your hand.

Strength
S1. Push-Ups or Modified Push-Ups—body
S4. Hips Raises—arms and shoulders

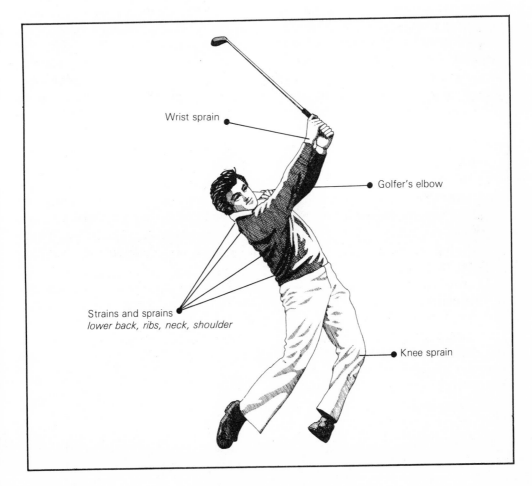

Wrist sprain

Golfer's elbow

Strains and sprains
lower back, ribs, neck, shoulder

Knee sprain

S5. Broomstick Rolls—wrists and hands
S6. Tennis Ball Squeeze—wrists and hands
S8. Fingertip Hip Raises—fingers
S16. Step-Ups—upper leg

Weight training under supervision: low-resistance, high-repetition exercises concentrating on back, shoulders, arms and wrists.

In addition, carry out swings using a shortened club—down to two foot—for wrist strengthening.

Also try holding the club in just the middle three fingers of the left hand (for right-handed players). This is an excellent exercise for strengthening wrist, forearm and fingers. It can be done at any time at home or in the office.

Heart and Lung
Running
Jogging
Swimming

HOME CIRCUIT
Preliminary warm-up
Ropework, if appropriate; otherwise jogging
F2. Trunk Twists
S1. Push-Ups or Modified Push-Ups
F13. Leg Swings
F3. Alternate Toe Touches
S16. Step-Ups
F7. Arm Circles
F11. The Lunge
S8. Fingertip Hip Raises

GOLF INJURIES
Golfer's Elbow: This is usually felt on the inside of the elbow, rather than the outside as in tennis elbow (see p. 132). It is usually due to a combination of overusing the muscles around the elbow during the follow-through of the swing and gripping the club too tightly. It is particularly prevalent in older golfers. For treatment, see tennis elbow. An effective remedial exercise is to lift a light weight, such as a bag containing a book, while seated, with the elbow resting on the arm of a chair. Frequent repetitions, starting with 10 and increasing to 25, are beneficial.

Knee Sprain: This is caused by the rotational action when driving and (particularly with older golfers) in walking over rough ground. The swing pattern can be at fault in the first instance and it is advisable to consult a coach.

Strains: Especially to lower back, ribs, neck and shoulder. These vary from nagging to acute and in most cases can be attributed to poor technique. See a golf pro. They are also caused by failure to warm up properly and failure to stretch the back and leg muscles thoroughly.

Wrist Strain: This is often due to taking too large a divot out of the ground, which jars the wrist. It can also lead to golfer's elbow.

Boxing

BOXING IS ONE OF the most physically exhausting of sports, even at the lowest levels. It calls primarily for a very high degree of stamina and general fitness, allied with all-round agility and footwork.

Specific fitness for boxing involves high heart and lung endurance; strength, particularly in the upper trunk, arms, wrists and legs; and flexibility, especially in the shoulders, waist, legs and arms. Flexibility is coming to be recognized as one of the most important attributes of the boxer, as it helps to lessen tension, which can have a disastrous effect on a boxer's performance in the ring.

Alternative Sports: Running, jogging, swimming, cycling and ropework are good for stamina building. Many trainers like to keep their young boxers together and encourage team games such as soccer, volleyball and basketball, all of which help general flexibility. Games for an individual include squash and badminton. Fencing is an excellent way of building trunk flexibility. The shot put and discus both require the same degree of nimble footwork and agility as the boxer.

Warm-Up: Warm-up before a bout or training session is extremely important and usually consists of some gentle jogging followed by flexibility exercises, especially for the neck and legs.

BOXING FITNESS EXERCISES
Flexibility
F1. Side Bends—hips and thighs
F2. Trunk Twists—trunk and neck
F3. Alternate Toe Touches—back, shoulders and arms
F4. Neck Rolls—neck
F7. Arm Circles—arms and upper trunk
F11. The Lunge—groin and thigh
F14. Knee Pulls—lower leg

Strength

S1. Push-Ups—body
S2. Pull-Ups—arms and shoulders
S3. Two-Chair Push-Ups—arms and shoulders
S5. Broomstick Rolls—wrists and hands
S10. Bent-Leg Sit-Ups—abdomen
S12. Squat Thrusts—thighs
S13. Sprinters—thighs
S16. Step-Ups—upper leg
S17. Bench Jumps—abdomen

In addition, weight training under supervision.

Heart and Lung

Running   Swimming
Jogging   Ropework

HOME CIRCUIT

Preliminary warm-up
Jogging on the spot
Ropework, if appropriate; otherwise jogging
S1. Push-Ups
F2. Trunk Twists
F11. The Lunge
S16. Step-Ups
F3. Alternate Toe Touches
F4. Neck Rolls
S12. Squat Thrusts

BOXING INJURIES

As in any contact sport, the incidence of injuries in boxing is high. Many of these occur in training rather than actually during a bout, and many strains

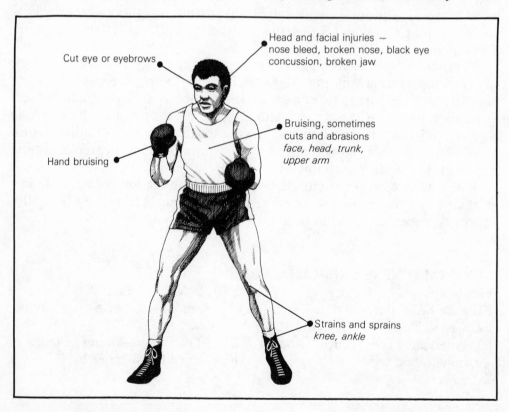

Cut eye or eyebrows

Hand bruising

Head and facial injuries —
nose bleed, broken nose, black eye
concussion, broken jaw

Bruising, sometimes
cuts and abrasions
*face, head, trunk,
upper arm*

Strains and sprains
knee, ankle

and sprains would be avoided if the boxer ensured that a full range of flexibility and strength exercises were carried out during general conditioning, as well as a thorough warm-up routine preceeding a workout or appearance in the ring.

Bruises, cuts and abrasions are common, particularly to the face, head, trunk and upper arms. **Cut eyes or eyebrows** can keep a boxer out of the ring for weeks. These could be serious and must be treated by a doctor immediately. Abrasions are most common on the leg or arm and are usually the result of falling and sliding on the canvas or scraping against the ring rope.

Other facial injuries include nosebleeds, broken noses, black eyes and cut lips (the latter often due to having ill-fitting gum shields), as well as other much more severe injuries. Fractured jaws are quite frequent in boxing, and concussion sometimes follows from a heavy blow to either the jaw or head. Most countries now have very strict rules about allowing a boxer back into the ring after having suffered concussion.

Fractures and severe bruising can also occur to the bones of the hand, despite protection afforded by bandaging under the gloves. Most vulnerable are the backs of the hands, the knuckles and thumbs.

In a sport in which footwork and agility are so important, **strains and sprains**, especially to the ankle and knee, are frequent, but flexibility and strengthening exercises for these parts of the body, combined with thorough warming-up, should do much to render them less likely.

Wrestling

WRESTLING REQUIRES MORE than pure strength, although strength, particularly in the upper trunk, is very important. The contest on the mat is one of move and countermove conducted at lightning speed and requiring instantaneous reaction. Stamina is essential in a wrestler, as is all-round body coordination and agility to counter surprise moves by an opponent.

Specific fitness for wrestling involves a high level of heart and lung endurance; strength in the upper body, legs and arms; and flexibility in the back and body, hips, legs and arms.

Alternative Sports: Running, jogging, swimming and weight training are all good stamina builders. Team games, such as soccer, rugby, football and field hockey, and racquet sports, especially tennis and squash, are good for body coordination and help speed the reactions. Gymnastics are excellent for general agility and for hip flexibility.

Warm-Up: In such an explosively muscular sport, the warm-up is all-important as a means of preventing muscle strains and also helping to create the right mental attitude for the contest. Wrestling warm-up is a highly individual matter and one with which wrestlers rapidly come to personal terms. The end result must be to bring the wrestler to peak physical and mental condition for an intensely exhausting period of 3-minute rounds during much of which he will be supporting a fair proportion of his opponent's weight as well as his own. Thus the limbs must be thoroughly supple and the whole body tuned up to be able to exert maximum strength at the outset, without fear of injury. Most wrestlers carry out some jogging, followed by a full range of flexibility exercises.

WRESTLING FITNESS EXERCISES

Flexibility

F1. Side Bends—hips and thighs
F2. Trunk Twists—trunk and neck
F3. Alternate Toe Touches—back, shoulders and arms
F7. Arm Circles—arms and upper body
F11. The Lunge—groin and thighs
F12. Hurdles—groin and thighs
F14. Knee Pulls—lower legs

Strength

Weight training, under supervision, is the most essential ingredient in wrestling fitness, and, when away from a gymnasium or other place of exercise with the necessary apparatus, most wrestlers improvise weight-training exercises at home.

Other valuable strength exercises are:

S1. Push-Ups—body
S2. Pull-Ups—arms and shoulders
S3. Two-Chair Push-Ups—arms and shoulders
S5. Broomstick Rolls—wrists and hands
S7. Fingertip Push-Ups—fingers
S10. Bent-Leg Sit-Ups—abdomen
S12. Squat Thrusts—thighs
S16. Step-Ups—upper leg
S17. Bench Jumps—upper leg
S19. Calf Raises—lower leg

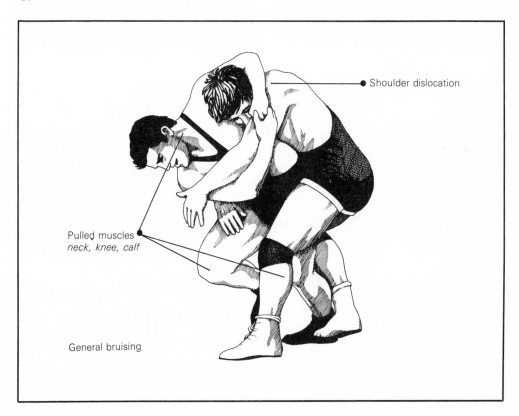

Shoulder dislocation

Pulled muscles
neck, knee, calf

General bruising

Heart and Lung

Running, including Fartlek and interval training. Sprints and shuttle runs are good for developing speed and reflexes.

Jogging

Swimming

Ropework: Jumping from the crouching position is excellent for heart and lung endurance, and also for leg and lower trunk strengthening.

HOME CIRCUIT

S1. Push-Ups
F2. Trunk Twists
S2. Pull-Ups
F3. Alternate Toe Touches
S10. Bent-Leg Sit-Ups
S3. Two-Chair Push-Ups
F12. Hurdles
F7. Arm Circles
S12. Squat Thrusts

WRESTLING INJURIES

Pulled muscles, especially in the neck, calf or knee, are the most prevalent wrestling injuries. These are most likely to occur at the start of a training session or contest, and are usually due to inadequate warm-up. Tension increases the likelihood and severity of injury, and until the newcomer to wrestling has found confidence in his own ability, he is quite likely to injure himself by falling on a too rigid arm or leg.

Fractures are rare, although dislocations, especially of the shoulder, do occur. These can usually be averted by proper conditioning and a thorough warm-up before a contest or training session.

Bruising is quite frequent, although seldom severe.

Fencing

FENCING IS A SPORT that is recommended by many authorities as both an all-round activity and one of the finest forms of physical and mental relaxation. As a sport, it requires a high degree of general fitness and considerable muscular and joint mobility. It also calls for footwork and body coordination of a very high order.

Specifically, fencing requires a high level of heart and lung endurance; strength, especially in the arm and upper body, as well as in the lower back, which is under considerable strain; and flexibility in the hips, legs, fingers and wrists.

Alternative Sports: Swimming and running are excellent for stamina building. Racquet games, especially tennis, squash and badminton, as well as basketball and volleyball are good for improving agility. Yoga is a fine form of general relaxation.

Warm-Up: Warming-up should include some gentle jogging followed by flexibility exercises. Then practice footwork and lunging.

FENCING EXERCISES
Flexibility
F1. Side Bends—hips and thighs
F2. Trunk Twists—trunk and neck
F3. Alternate Toe Touches—back, shoulders and arms
F7. Arm Circles—arms and upper trunk
F9. Wrist Shakes—wrists
F11. The Lunge—groin and thigh
F14. Knee Pulls—lower leg
F15. Calf Stretches—lower leg

Strength
S1. Push-Ups or Modified Push-Ups —body
S2. Pull-Ups—arms and shoulders
S5. Broomstick Rolls—arms and shoulders
S6. Tennis Ball Squeeze variation—wrist and hands (use a squash ball and squeeze between thumb and forefinger)
S8. Fingertip Hip Raises—fingers
S16. Step-Ups—upper legs

In addition, weight training under supervision: low-resistance high-repetition exercises with emphasis on arms, upper body and lower back.

Heart and Lung
Running
Swimming
Ropework

HOME CIRCUIT
Ropework, if appropriate; otherwise jogging
S1. Push-Ups or Modified Push-Ups
F1. Side Bends
S16. Step-Ups
F11. The Lunge

S2. Pull-Ups
F14. Knee Pulls
S8. Fingertip Hip Raises
F15. Calf Stretches

FENCING INJURIES
Bruises: These are usually due to off-target hits and are especially common on the forearm (foil and saber) and shoulder (all weapons). The sword hand is also subject to bruising by a heavy blow (this can also lead to finger breaks).

  Strains and Sprains: Hamstring pulls, often caused by slipping on poor floors, are sometimes made more likely by imbalance between the relative mus-

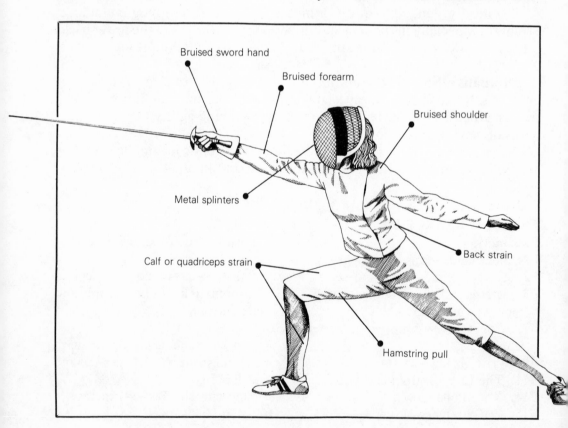

cle strengths of the quadriceps at the front of the thigh and the hamstrings at the back. This can be remedied by balanced strength and flexibility exercises. In addition, the lunge can cause strain in the quadriceps muscles or the calf. Flexibility and strength exercises during the conditioning program and a thorough warm-up should do much toward lessening the likelihood of these injuries.

Metal Splinters: These are caused by sword clash, especially with the saber. To extract metal splinters a strong magnet will usually suffice.

Should a splinter penetrate the mask and get into the eye, immediate medical attention is essential.

Back Strain: This is especially evident at waist level and is due to constant twisting. If mild, a hot bath or shower will ease the discomfort; if persistent or more severe, a doctor should be consulted, as disc trouble could be indicated.

A Note on Mask Care: The protection provided by the mask is essential in fencing. This should be inspected regularly; in particular look out for rusting in the area of the nose and mouth.

Judo

JUDO IS AS MUCH A philosophy as it is a modern combat sport. Derived from the ancient Japanese ju-jitsu style of fighting, judo basically requires skill coupled with power and suppleness. It is recognized as an excellent physical training activity for developing both general fitness and stamina. In addition, a number of athletes take up judo as an aid to body coordination and to speed up their reactions, as well as to teach themselves how to fall in their own sport without injury.

Physically, judo contests demand short bursts of explosive effort during a 3–20-minute period. It therefore requires a basic level of heart and lung endurance, although this will develop with practice in the sport; strength, particularly in the upper and lower body and legs; and flexibility in the body and legs.

Alternative Sports: Running, swimming, cycling and jogging are all good stamina builders. Racquet sports such as squash, badminton and racquetball help to improve body coordination and general flexibility, as do basketball, volleyball and handball.

Warm-Up: The warm-up in judo is essential; otherwise muscle strains and sprains are certain to ensue. Carry out a little jogging followed by flexibility exercises, with emphasis on the body, both upper and lower, and the leg muscles.

JUDO FITNESS EXERCISES
Flexibility
F1. Side Bends—hips and thighs
F2. Trunk Twists—trunk and neck
F3. Alternate Toe Touches—back, shoulders and arms

F7. Arm Circles—arms and upper body
F11. The Lunge—groin and thighs
F12. Hurdles—groin and thighs
F15. Calf Stretches—lower legs

Strength

S1. Push-Ups or Modified Push-Ups
   —body
S2. Pull-Ups—arms and shoulders
S9. "Bicycling"—abdomen
S10. Bent-Leg Sit-Ups—abdomen
S12. Squat Thrusts—thighs
S16. Step-Ups—upper leg
S17. Bench Jumps—upper leg

In addition, an excellent exercise for judo players is the **Cat Dip:** Adopt a position as shown, with feet well apart and hands outstretched. Bring the head and shoulders forward in a low swooping movement, then reverse the movement until the former position is adopted. This is an excellent flexibility and strength exercise for the back and trunk, and is also useful for general body suppling. Repeated a number of times, it is also a good exercise for stamina building. However, it should only be practiced by the already fit.

Repetitions: 5, increasing to 10

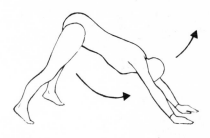

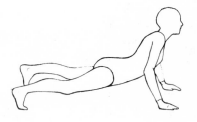

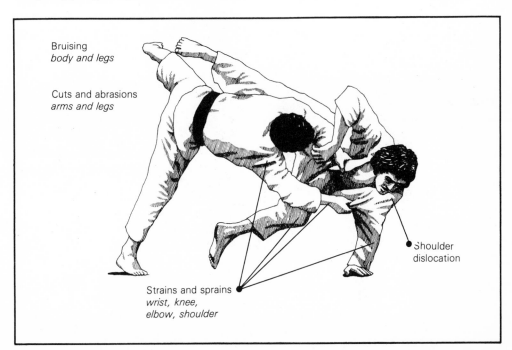

Bruising
body and legs

Cuts and abrasions
arms and legs

Shoulder
dislocation

Strains and sprains
*wrist, knee,
elbow, shoulder*

Heart and Lung

Running, particularly Fartlek, interval
   and sprint training (10–15 yards
   maximum)
Jogging
Ropework (also good for footwork)
Swimming

HOME CIRCUIT

Preliminary warm-up
Jogging on the spot
Ropework, if appropriate
F2. Trunk Twists
S1. Push-Ups or Modified Push-Ups
F11. The Lunge
F15. Calf Stretches
F7. Arm Circles
S10. Bent-Leg Sit-Ups
S2. Pull-Ups
S12. Squat Thrusts

JUDO INJURIES

These usually arise through falling incorrectly. The most frequent judo injury is **bruising** particularly to the body or legs.

Cuts and abrasions are also quite common, the arms and legs being the most vulnerable here.

Strains and sprains: The wrist, knee, elbow and shoulder (which is also occasionally subject to dislocation) are most vulnerable. The likelihood of injury can be minimized with proper strength and flexibility exercises and a really thorough warm-up before a training session or match.

Karate

KARATE IS A COMBAT sport of Chinese origin, unlike judo and aikido which derive from the ancient Japanese ju-jitsu style of fighting. It is generally recognized as the most forceful of the martial arts and involves striking, blocking and thrusting, using the head, elbows, forearms and knees as well as the hands and feet to defeat an opponent. The karate-ka, or player, requires some strength, but primarily speed, agility and lightning-quick reflexes, for the karate blow is fast (it has been estimated that it is traveling at a speed of over 20 feet per second) and can break a concrete slab 4 inches thick.

Specific fitness for karate calls for some heart and lung endurance with specific strength in the trunk, arms and legs, but this must not be at the expense of flexibility. General suppleness is all-important in karate, especially in the trunk, shoulders, hips, arms, wrists and upper and lower legs.

Alternative Sports: Running, walking, swimming and ropework are all good for stamina building. Racquet sports, particularly squash and badminton, as well as basketball and volleyball are good for developing hand/eye and general body coordination. Gymnastics is excellent for overall suppleness.

Warm-Up: The warm-up is crucial in karate and extensive warm-up sessions are an integral part of the sport. These include a series of flexibility exercises designed to supple the whole body and can last for up to 20 minutes. The emphasis, however, should be on the pelvis and abdomen, hamstrings and legs in order to get the necessary "snap" which is the hallmark of the good karate player.

KARATE FITNESS EXERCISES
Flexibility
F1. Side Bends—hips and thighs

F2. Trunk Twists—trunk and neck

F3. Alternate Toe Touches—back, shoulders and arms

F4. Neck Rolls—neck

F10. The Reach—abdomen, thigh and calf

F11. The Lunge—groin and thighs

F12. Hurdles—groin and thighs

F14. Knee Pulls—lower leg

Strength
S1. Push-Ups or Modified Push-Ups —body

S2. Pull-Ups—arms and shoulders

S3. Two-Chair Push-Ups—arms and shoulders

S5. Broomstick Rolls—wrists, hands

S8. Fingertip Hip Raises—fingers

S10. Bent-Leg Sit-Ups—abdomen

S13. Sprinters—upper legs

S17. Bench Jumps—abdomen

In addition, **Cat Dips** (*see* Judo, p. 121) is an excellent flexibility and strength exercise for the back, as well as a good stamina builder.

Knuckle toughening is usually done against a *makiwara*, a straw-covered post.

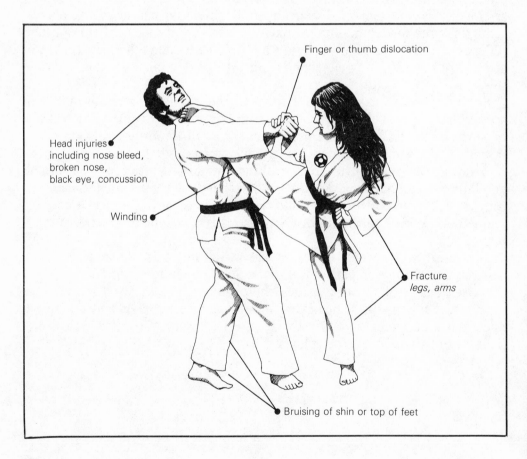

Finger or thumb dislocation

Head injuries including nose bleed, broken nose, black eye, concussion

Winding

Fracture *legs, arms*

Bruising of shin or top of feet

Heart and Lung
Running
Jogging
Walking
Swimming
Ropework

HOME CIRCUIT
Preliminary warm-up
Jogging on the spot
Ropework, if appropriate; otherwise
 jogging
S1. Push-ups
F2. Trunk Twists
F12. Hurdles
S16. Step-Ups
F3. Alternate Toe Touches
S10. Bent-Leg Sit-Ups
F4. Neck Rolls
S13. Sprinters

KARATE INJURIES
The target sites in karate embrace the head, face and trunk, so there is wide scope for injury. The head, face and neck are the most commonly injured, next in frequency are the limbs and finally the trunk itself.

Injuries to the head and face include **bruising, cuts, abrasions, lost teeth, black eyes,** and **bleeding** or **broken noses. Concussion** can occur, especially if a player hits the floor with his head.

The fingers and thumb may suffer dislocation in a fall, but the most common injuries to the limbs are to the feet, caused either in kicking or in blocking a kick. This can cause **bruising,** especially to the shin or the top of the foot. Ice and rest would seem to be the most satisfactory treatment for this injury, but flexibility and strength exercises for the foot would help a lot.

Fractures do occur, usually due to a blocked kick and most commonly to the leg and arm.

Winding, due to a blow to the solar plexus, also occurs.

Many of these injuries can be prevented by wearing gum shields, groin guards, fist and foot pads and a protective helmet, but some traditional karate enthusiasts oppose such refinements.

Aikido

AIKIDO IS A SPORT that is gaining in popularity, both as a competitive game and as a fine means of general exercise and promoting physical well-being. In addition, a growing number of athletes in other sports are looking at aikido as an excellent way of improving suppleness and speeding the reflexes and reactions. Although less physical than judo, aikido is also derived from the ancient Japanese ju-jitsu style of fighting. It is a purely defensive form of martial art involving first avoiding attack and then neutralizing the attacker.

Aikido relies on good posture, balance and timing, in particular for taking advantage of an assailant's own impetus and turning it to the defender's advantage. Unlike judo, it is largely conducted at arm's length; the body is hardly brought into play at all.

Specifically, aikido needs some heart and lung endurance; strength in the arms and wrists as well as the legs; and flexibility in all parts of the body, especially the shoulders, arms, wrists and legs.

Alternative Sports: Jogging, swimming and running are all good for stamina building. Best of all is ropework, which adds to the general suppleness of the body and aids footwork. Racquet sports, such as squash and badminton, and basketball and volleyball (both of which involve a lot of back muscle work as well as wrist flexibility) are also beneficial. Other good alternatives are gymnastics (for general suppleness) and yoga (for physical and mental relaxation).

Warm-Up: The warm-up in aikido is crucial and usually consists of a 30- to 40-minute series of general flexibility exercises designed to limber up as well as relax the body and aid concentration.

AIKIDO FITNESS EXERCISES
Flexibility
F1. Side Bends—hips and thighs

F2. Trunk Twists—trunk and neck

F3. Alternate Toe Touches—back, shoulders and arms

F4. Neck Rolls—neck

F6. Wing Stretchers—shoulders

F8. Arm Flings—arms and upper trunk

F9. Wrist Shakes—wrists and hands

F11. The Lunge—groin and thighs

F14. Knee Pulls—lower legs

Strength
S1. Push-Ups or Modified Push-Ups —body

S2. Pull-Ups—arms and shoulders

S5. Broomstick Rolls—wrists and hands

S6. Tennis Ball Squeeze—wrists and hands

S8. Fingertip Hip Raises—fingers

S11. Half Squats—thighs

S16. Step-Ups—upper leg

S17. Bench Jumps–lower leg

In addition, weight training under supervision. This should not be at the expense of flexibility. Carry out low-resistance, high-repetition exercises, especially for the arms, wrists and legs.

Heart and Lung
Running	Swimming
Jogging	Ropework

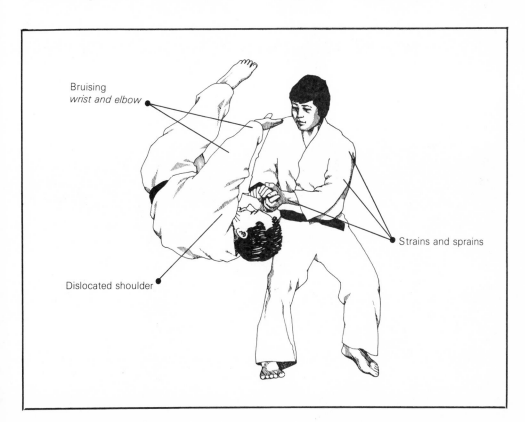

Bruising *wrist and elbow*

Strains and sprains

Dislocated shoulder

HOME CIRCUIT
Preliminary warm-up

Ropework, if appropriate; otherwise jogging

F4. Neck Rolls

S1. Push-Ups or Modified Push-Ups

F2. Trunk Twists

S8. Fingertip Hip Raises

F3. Alternate Toe Touches

F8. Arm Flings

S16. Step-Ups

F1. Side Bends

S17. Bench Jumps

AIKIDO INJURIES
Injuries in aikido are usually due to poor conditioning and/or tension, which is especially common with beginners. The nature of the throw and fall in aikido can cause injury—particularly to the arms, wrists and shoulders—until the player has learned how to fall properly, which is quite essential to the art of the sport.

Bruises, particularly to the wrists and elbow, do occur.

Strains and sprains are the most frequent injuries. These are usually to the elbow, wrist and shoulder (which, occasionally, may also become dislocated). Flexibility and strength exercises for these parts of the body, combined with a really thorough warm-up, should do much to avoid these injuries.

Tennis

TENNIS FITNESS IS A much-neglected aspect of the game. Most occasional tennis players go on court and with only a short preliminary rally launch off into a highly energetic game. Few realize just how physically exacting tennis is, and how much their standard of play would improve if they took a little trouble over their general fitness.

Tennis requires considerable stamina and speed to get around the court, as well as specific strength and nimble footwork. It ideally calls for an all-year-round conditioning program, but few players carry this out. Speed in tennis, as with other racquet sports, is not the straight-ahead speed of the sprinter; the game involves short dashes forward, backward and sideways, and this frequent change of direction and stop-start action throws tremendous strain on the lower limbs.

In addition, today's power game puts considerable stress on the muscles of arm, shoulder and back, and new court surfaces have increased the risk of injuries to the knee and ankle.

The true tennis player must be supremely fit. It is only necessary to watch a two-hour championship match taking place under full sun to understand the physical drain imposed on a player and to see how quickly a less fit player tires. As fatigue sets in, the muscles tighten and the risks of injury become greater.

Specifically, tennis demands a high degree of heart and lung endurance. Strength is required in the upper body, shoulders, back, arms and legs; and flexibility is called for in the shoulder, elbow, wrists, hips, knees and ankles.

Alternative Sports: Jogging, running, swimming, squash, badminton, bicycling, soccer and basketball are good alternative or off-season sports, but most tennis players believe that more tennis is the best—and only—conditioner for the game.

Warm-Up: Many tennis injuries are due to inadequate warm-up. Unlike many other games, tennis requires explosive bursts of energy right from the start of play (e.g., the opening service). If the muscles and the body generally are not properly warmed up, muscle pulls and other injuries are far more likely to occur. Yet how often does one see only a short practice rally or two as the sole limbering-up process—especially on club courts reserved for a limited period. It is far better to have a briefer match and enjoy it more with less chance of injury, than to blast off without proper warm-up. This is especially important during cold weather and with older players because muscles tighten with cold and age. Warm-up should take place with sweaters or sweat suits still on and should continue to the point of sweating.

Pregame warm-up should include some jogging followed by flexibility exercises, which can be carried out off court. In addition, either on court or at the side of the court, practice forehand and backhand ground strokes slowly and rhythmically with the racquet cover still on to give extra air resistance. Bouncing the ball on alternate sides of the racquet—which involves turning over the wrist—not only helps flex the wrist muscles but improves hand/eye coordination.

Pregame Practice: This is the ideal time to stretch the muscles slowly while executing actual shots—especially overhead shots (serve and smash), which place great strain on back, shoulders and arms.

The pregame practice also gives the player a chance to get the feel of the court, assess the bounce of the ball, test opponents and discover their weaknesses, and generally unwind so the game can be approached in a relaxed state.

TENNIS EXERCISES
Flexibility
F1. Side Bends—hips and thighs
F2. Trunk Twists—trunk and neck
F4. Neck Rolls—neck
F5. Shoulder Shrugs—shoulders
F7. Arm Circles—arms and upper body
F12. The Lunge—groin and thighs
F15. Calf Stretches—lower legs

Strength
S1. Push-Ups or Modified Push-Ups —body
S2. Pull-Ups—arms and shoulders
S5. Broomstick Rolls—wrists and hands

S6. Tennis Ball Squeeze—wrists and hands
S9. "Bicycling"—abdomen
S12. Squat Thrusts—thighs
S16. Step-Ups—upper legs
S17. Bench Jumps—upper legs
S19. Calf Raises—lower legs

Weight training under supervision: low-resistance, high-repetition exercises, with emphasis on the upper body, shoulders, back, arms and legs.

In addition, practice the **Newspaper Crumble:** Hold the corner of a page of a newspaper in the racquet hand and slowly crumble it. Carry out the exercise with the palm upward. Then take another page and repeat the exercise with the palm downward.

Heart and Lung
Running, especially Fartlek and interval training, shuttle runs and zigzags. Uphill and sandhill running are excellent for increasing leg strength
Jogging
Swimming
Ropework

HOME CIRCUIT
Preliminary warm-up
Ropework, if appropriate; otherwise jogging

S1. Push-Ups or Modified Push-Ups
F2. Trunk Twists
F12. The Lunge
F4. Neck Rolls
S10. Bent-Leg Sit-Ups
S16. Step-Ups
F7. Arm Circles
S17. Bench Jumps
F1. Side Bends
S12. Squat Thrusts

Improvisation: Practice tennis strokes with a large frying pan. Passing a bucket or pail containing a few books or water from hand to hand with a rhythmic swing from the hips is an excellent flexibility exercise.

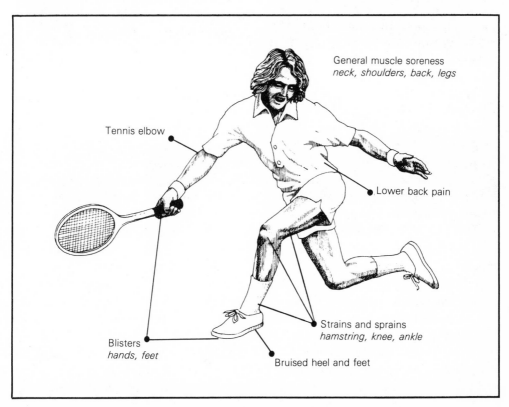

General muscle soreness
neck, shoulders, back, legs

Tennis elbow

Lower back pain

Strains and sprains
hamstring, knee, ankle

Blisters
hands, feet

Bruised heel and feet

TENNIS INJURIES

Tennis Elbow: The causes of tennis elbow are many and varied, and by no means are they all associated with tennis (in tennis, however, it is more common with players over 35). Anatomically, tennis elbow is an inflammation of the attachments of the forearm muscles to the outer side of the elbow, which is aggravated by frequent shocks as the ball hits the racquet.

In tennis the usual cause is incorrect technique, usually in the form of hitting the ball with the elbow bent (which causes the forearm muscles to take most of the impact) and not transferring the weight of the body through the shoulder when striking the ball. Beginners often lead with the elbow when they play their shots rather than pointing the elbow toward the ground which, in mechanical terms, is the way to avoid undue strain on forearm and elbow. Leading with the elbow can also occur when the player gets too close to or overruns the ball; this then requires the execution of a scoop-like shot— especially on the backhand—which places great strain on the forearm.

When played late, the forehand volley or ground stroke requires greater wrist action than is advisable. Sliced or topspin shots on the backhand or forehand also put strain on the wrist and forearm. The change from a slow to a faster surface can throw out a player's timing and cause the ball to be taken late. Similarly, using a heavier ball than usual or balls that have become wet and heavy can contribute to tennis elbow.

In serving, tennis elbow is aggravated by mistiming, often due to the body weight coming forward too soon, leaving the arm to catch up. This means that on impact the arm and racquet are at the wrong angle, which results in a low trajectory that places considerable strain on the whole arm, in particular on the forearm and wrist. The server in fact is then serving with the arm only, rather than properly using the weight of the body. Heavily spun services can also aggravate tennis elbow.

Symptoms: A growing pain and tenderness, usually on the outer side of the elbow and upper forearm, but sometimes extending down toward the wrist. It is extremely painful to extend the elbow fully. Occasionally tennis elbow is felt on the inside of the elbow and at times extends to the shoulder.

Treatment: Tennis elbow usually clears up after a few months, providing total rest can be given. This not only precludes taking part in any sport that might aggravate the condition, but also means avoiding lifting any heavy weights in everyday life—such as boxes, suitcases, buckets of water—or even having your hand shaken too violently.

On first feeling tennis elbow, it is advisable to stop playing immediately. Application of ice eases the discomfort. If very painful it could be worth putting on a sling to discourage moving the arm.

There are several other ways of alleviating tennis elbow enough to be able to play. The use of a brace or elasticized bandage placed at the top of the forearm below the elbow is of considerable assistance; others find a wrist strap more effective still. Changing to a racquet with a lighter grip or a lighter head may also make tennis elbow less painful. Check that the racquet is not strung too tightly; the tighter the stringing, the greater the jarring effect when hitting the ball (50 to 54 pounds of tension is ideal). Gut is believed to be easier on the elbow than nylon.

Most tennis-elbow sufferers agree that a wider grip eases the pain, although there are those that advocate a thinner grip. The handle must not be too large, though, or else it can lead to blisters on the playing hand and tired forearm muscles. The greater flexibility of metal over wood racquets also takes some of the jarring effect out of a shot.

Professional treatment for chronic tennis elbow varies from injections to deep massage to immobilization in plaster or ultrasonic therapy.

Prevention: Tennis elbow is principally due to incorrect stroking, and for this there is no better preventative than correct coaching. However, here are a few general points:

- Always warm-up fully with off-court exercise and a pre-game rally. Particularly concentrate on exercising the playing arm and shoulder with overhead shots.
- Take the ball when it is in front of the lead foot rather than when it has passed.
- Hold the racquet loosely in the hand until the moment of contact.

- Play the backhand with elbow straight, leading with the shoulder rather than with the forearm. The two-handed backhand takes the strain off the normal playing arm. Two-handed players don't seem to suffer from tennis elbow, but the loss of reach must be compensated for by greater mobility.
- Work on wrist and arm flexibility and strength exercises (*see* Part I).

Blisters on Hands: Playing will harden the hands. Dabbing with alcohol or a skin-hardening agent will also help. It is important to use a correctly sized grip and a dry handle. Be sure to wipe hands and handle when necessary. If you are a constant sufferer, it may be necessary to wear a glove on the playing hand.

Feet: Talcum powder on the feet before play helps prevent foot blisters. Harden the feet with alcohol or skin-hardening agent. Many players wear two pairs of socks.

General Muscle Soreness: Particularly in the neck, shoulders, back and legs. A hot bath or shower and gentle massage or kneading under water helps to relieve this. For older players, flexibility exercises while in the bath or shower eases the muscles after play and helps prevent stiffness afterward. Sauna, massage or swimming in a heated pool are all beneficial.

Strains and Sprains: Especially to hamstrings, knees and ankles. These are becoming increasingly common with the introduction of new kinds of court surfaces, which tend to prevent the natural slide of the foot.

Apply ice, and rest. Strains and sprains may take two weeks or more to heal—the older the person, the longer the healing time. It is important to return to sport gradually; as a muscle will shorten while healing, carry out gentle flexibility exercises when ready. Do not, on any account, hurry the process. In the longer term, set about strengthening exercises.

Warming up thoroughly is very important in preventing strains and sprains. Wearing the correct sole for the type of playing surface is crucial; many modern composition surfaces make a more slippery sole advisable.

Lower Back Pain: This is due to constant stooping for low balls and straining during the service. It can also be caused by not changing out of wet and sweaty tennis clothes after play. This can lead to chills in the lumbar region; the crucial areas are where constriction of the clothing occurs, e.g., at the waist.

Rest for 7–10 days from tennis or other exercise which places strain upon the back. Return to the game slowly and gradually and carry out flexibility and strengthening exercises when recovered.

Bruised Heels and Feet: Apply ice and rest if the bruising is severe. In most cases it is usually enough to get shoes with more sole padding, raised heels and good arch support.

Squash

SQUASH IS A VIGOROUS SPORT that involves a great deal of intensive exercise in a short time. A highly popular pursuit among part-time athletes (and one which is being adopted by more and more people every year), it is an excellent all-round conditioner. Newcomers to the game should note that it demands a reasonable degree of general fitness before starting to play, for squash is a start-stop sport requiring great agility, speed of movement and considerable stamina. It also calls for good body coordination, excellent footwork and ball control of a high order.

Specific fitness for squash involves a high level of heart and lung endurance; strength in stomach, back, shoulders, arms, wrists and legs; and flexibility in the body, arms, wrists and upper and lower legs.

Alternative Sports: Badminton, volleyball, cricket, baseball and skiing (both snow and water) are good alternative sports; also running, swimming and cycling, which are useful for building stamina. But the best conditioner for squash is more squash.

Warm-Up: The problem with the warm-up in squash is that courts are often in such high demand that many players, conscious of their limited time, are reluctant to warm-up at all. As a result they throw themselves straight into the game before their bodies are properly tuned. The consequence is inevitable injury, even if the player has a high degree of prior fitness.

A warm-up of some sort is essential in squash and can usually be achieved before going on court. If convenient, a gentle jog to the court, rather than a walk, is a good beginning to the limbering-up process. After changing, do a few stretching exercises and flexibility exercises (particularly for the shoulder, neck, back, hamstrings and calves), and utilize every moment before play. The pregame practice offers a number of opportunities, namely:

- To break yourself in slowly and gently, warming and stretching the muscles as you do so.

- To assess the court (lighting, background, height of ceiling, type of floor, etc.) and the bounce of the ball.
- To assess your opponent's strengths and weaknesses, while at the same time trying to ensure that your own strokes are in good working order.

SQUASH FITNESS EXERCISES

Flexibility

F2. Trunk Twists—trunk and neck

F3. Alternate Toe Touches—back, shoulder and arms

F4. Neck Rolls—neck

F7. Arm Circles—arms and upper body

F11. The Lunge—groin and thigh

F14. Knee Pulls—lower leg

Strength

S1. Push-Ups or Modified Push-Ups —body

S2. Pull-Ups—arms and shoulders

S6. Tennis Ball Squeeze—wrists and hands

S10. Bent-Leg Sit-Ups—abdomen

S15. Leg Raises—upper leg

S16. Step-Ups—upper leg

S19. Calf Raises—lower leg

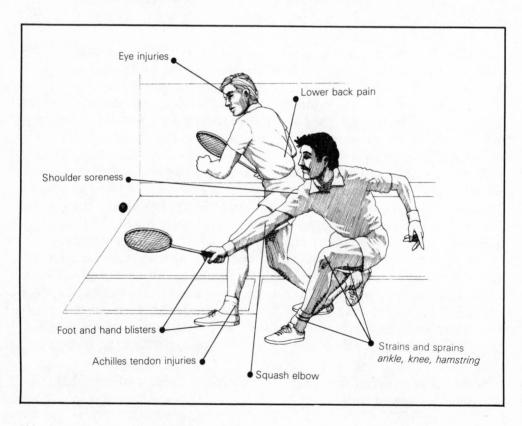

In addition, weight training under supervision is beneficial, particularly low-resistance high-repetition exercises with emphasis on abdomen, back, shoulders, arms, wrists and legs.

Heart and Lung

Running on the spot—high step (bring the knee right up to the chest).

Running, especially Fartlek and interval training, zigzag running and sprint training; also backward running.

On-Court Running: Squash requires quick movements of short duration and covering short distances; runs should be of no more than 15 seconds, with 15-second rests, for no longer than a total of 5 minutes.

The design and floor lines of a squash court offer many combinations of these basic forms of on-court exercise.

Ropework

Cycling

HOME CIRCUIT

Preliminary warm-up

Jogging on the spot

Ropework if appropriate: otherwise jogging

S1. Push-Ups or Modified Push-Ups

F2. Trunk Twists

S2. Pull-Ups

F11. The Lunge

S16. Step-Ups

F3. Alternate Toe Touches

S10. Bent-Leg Sit-Ups

F7. Arm Circles

SQUASH INJURIES

Blisters (hands and feet): These are a common complaint with squash players. It is a good idea to harden the hands and feet with alcohol or a skin-hardening agent. Shoes should fit properly, particularly at the sides and top.

Lower Back Pain: Brought about either by the player's constant stooping or an awkward twist or turn. It is a complaint that frequently afflicts even the fittest of squash players, and it can cause constant and recurring trouble unless treated properly at the outset. It is advisable to see a doctor. Resting on a hard mattress or bedboard with a pillow under the knees may be helpful.

Shoulder Soreness: This often occurs when a player has skimped the warm-up. It usually wears off after a few days' rest. Heat treatment after 48 hours is beneficial.

Squash Elbow: A common squash complaint, this is usually felt just above the elbow (rather than below it as in tennis elbow), and is often due to incorrect technique or too much practice at the same shot.

For treatment, *see* Tennis, pp. 132–133. It could help to have a coach check your stroke production; you may not be keeping up the head of the racquet. A thicker grip sometimes eases the pain, as does an elastic bandage or brace just below the elbow. Nothing can make up for complete rest from the game until the condition has worn off.

Strains and Sprains: Particularly to ankle, knee or hamstring. These are often caused when the forward foot slips while the player is lunging forward to retrieve a ball. Make sure that the soles of your shoes are in good condition.

Twists and turns can also cause **knee injuries,** which can vary from mild sprains to torn cartilages. Knee-strengthening and flexibility exercises, plus a really thorough warm-up before play, should make these less likely.

Bruised heels: Another common squash injury, which can be very uncomfortable. Make sure your shoes have ample sole padding and raised inner heels. Plastic heel cups also help.

Achilles Tendon Injuries: These vary from mild irritation to partial or even complete rupture. The latter often results in a noise like a pistol shot, and the player feels as though he has been hit hard at the back of the leg.

With the squash racquet traveling through the air at 90mph and the ball itself nearer 100mph, the possibility of serious **eye injury** is very high. Increasing concern is being felt in the squash world about the risk of eye injury, and eye guards and protectors are becoming more frequent on court. Care and quick reflexes are really the only true preventatives, but for those who wear glasses the dangers are more considerable. It is essential to wear glasses with safety lenses and sturdy rims. To avoid them being knocked off, tie glasses on with string or elastic. If you can wear them, contact lenses, especially soft ones, are a good bet.

Badminton

BADMINTON IS PLAYED at a tremendous pace and requires very fast reactions. It involves a lot of running and demands both explosive bursts of speed for short distances and lightning changes of direction. Much of the game is played in a half-squat position, which in itself is physically exhausting. Also, as the badminton player must reach higher and lower than in either squash or tennis, it calls for great suppleness, especially in the trunk.

Specific fitness for badminton involves a high standard of all-round conditioning with excellent heart and lung endurance; strength, especially in the trunk and abdomen, arms and legs; and flexibility in the trunk and back, shoulders, arms and legs.

Alternative Sports: The essential start-stop movement and hand/eye coordination needed in badminton is found in most racquet games, and many badminton players are enthusiastic squash and tennis players. Running, cycling and swimming are excellent for stamina building.

Warm-Up: This is an essential ingredient of the game and usually consists of a little gentle jogging and flexibility exercises. Some players do these on a regular day-to-day basis as part of their general conditioning routine.

BADMINTON FITNESS EXERCISES

Flexibility
F2. Trunk Twists—trunk and neck
F3. Alternate Toe Touches—back, shoulders and arms
F4. Neck Rolls—neck
F7. Arm Circles—arms and upper body
F9. Wrist Shakes—wrists and hands

F11. The Lunge—groin and thigh
F12. Hurdles—groin and thigh

Strength
S1. Push-ups or Modified Push-Ups —body
S3. Two-Chair Push-Ups—arms and shoulders

S5. Broomstick Rolls—wrists and hands

S10. Bent-Leg Sit-Ups—abdomen

S11. Half Squats—thighs

S12. Squat Thrusts—thighs

S16. Step-Ups—upper leg

S19. Calf Raises—lower leg

In addition, weight training under supervision: low-resistance, high-repetition exercises with emphasis on trunk, abdomen, shoulders, arms and legs.

Heart and Lung

Running, in particular Fartlek and interval training are good, as are sprint training and shuttle runs; on-court sequence training—running backwards, forwards and from side to side—is also popular

Jogging

Ropework (also excellent for improving footwork and body coordination)

HOME CIRCUIT

Preliminary warm-up

Jogging on the spot

Ropework, if appropriate; otherwise jogging

S1. Push-Ups or Modified Push-Ups

F4. Neck Rolls

S16. Step-Ups

F2. Trunk Twists

S3. Two-Chair Push-Ups

F7. Arm Circles

S12. Squat Thrusts

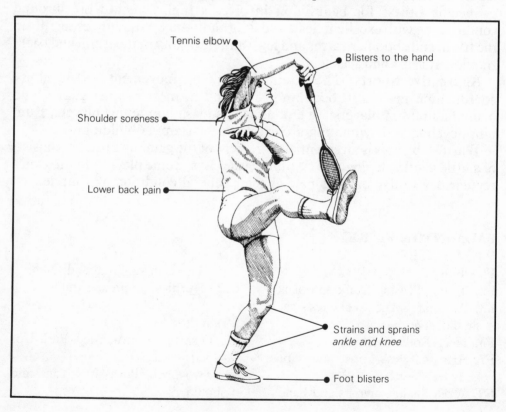

Tennis elbow

Blisters to the hand

Shoulder soreness

Lower back pain

Strains and sprains
ankle and knee

Foot blisters

BADMINTON INJURIES

Blisters: Both to hands and feet. These are one of the most frequent badminton injuries. It is well worth setting out at the start of the season to harden both hands and feet, using alcohol or a skin-hardening agent. Also make sure that shoes fit properly, particularly at the sides and top.

Falls lead to **general bruising** of the body, the upper arms and legs being most susceptible. Occasionally, falls can lead to fractures of fingers or thumb, when a player puts out a hand to break a fall.

Muscle soreness: Particularly of the shoulder. This is quite a common condition, especially if a player skimps on warming-up. It usually wears off after a few days' rest. Heat treatment and hot baths after 48 hours are also beneficial.

Pain in the lower back: This is a frequent badminton injury brought about by constantly stooping to play a shot. It is aggravated by the half-squat position adopted for a lot of the game, and can also be caused by turning awkwardly or by smashing. Even the fittest badminton players are subject to lower back pain, and it can cause constant and recurring trouble unless properly treated at the first sign. It is advisable to see a doctor. Resting on a hard mattress or bed board with a pillow under the knees may be helpful.

Sprains and Strains: Particularly of the knees and ankles. These may be caused by awkward twists and turns. Proper conditioning and a really thorough warm-up should do a lot to lessen the chance of these happening. Playing shoes must be in good condition to prevent slipping on court.

Tennis Elbow: A condition that is becoming more prevalent in high-class badminton due to current power-play techniques, which require the elbow to be bent rather than straight when executing a shot. Awkward back-of-the-court shots also contribute to the onset of tennis elbow. The condition in badminton is similar to squash elbow, in that the pain is usually felt above the elbow, badminton players, however, tend to refer to this complaint as "tennis" elbow.

Arm and wrist-strengthening exercises will help in the avoidance of tennis elbow. A change of grip is often beneficial, as is an elbow brace (*see* p. 133). In chronic cases, the root cause may be bad technique, in which case it is advisable to see a coach.

Racquetball

RACQUETBALL AS A PASTIME requires no fitness at all; at a higher, more competitive level, it is an immensely demanding and excitingly offensive sport. For children, it is an ideal introduction to other racquet sports.

As a high-speed sport, racquetball calls more specifically for a high level of heart and lung endurance; strength, particularly in the arms, legs, wrists and trunk; and flexibility in the lower leg, arms and wrists.

Alternative Sports: Running, jogging, cycling and swimming are good for general stamina building. Other racquet sports, basketball and volleyball are useful in improving general ball control.

Warm-Up: The warm-up in racquetball is important and usually consists of some off-court jogging and stretching before the game, and then a pregame warm-up on court.

RACQUETBALL FITNESS EXERCISES

Flexibility

F2. Trunk Twists—trunk and neck

F3. Alternate Toe Touches—back, shoulders and arms

F4. Neck Rolls—neck

F7. Arm Circles—arms and upper body

F9. Wrist Shakes—wrists

F11. The Lunge—groin and thighs

F14. Knee Pulls—lower legs

Strength

S1. Push-Ups or Modified Push-Ups —body

S2. Pull-Ups—arms and shoulders

S5. Broomstick Rolls—wrists, hands

S6. Tennis Ball Squeeze—wrists and hands

S10. Bent-Leg Sit-Ups—abdomen

S16. Step-Ups—upper legs

S19. Calf Raises—lower legs

In addition, weight training under supervision: low-resistance, high-repetition exercises, especially for arms and wrists, legs and back.

Heart and Lung
Running, especially Fartlek and interval training, shuttle runs and zigzags

Jogging   Swimming
Ropework   Cycling

HOME CIRCUIT
Preliminary warm-up
Jogging in Place
Ropework, if appropriate, otherwise jogging

S1. Push-Ups or Modified Push-ups
F2. Trunk Twists
F11. The Lunge
S2. Pull-Ups
F7. Arm Circles
S10. Bent-Leg Sit-Ups
F3. Alternate Toe Touches
S16. Step-Ups

RACQUETBALL INJURIES
At lower levels of participation, racquetball injuries are neither frequent nor severe. However at more intensive and competitive levels a number of injuries do occur.

Blisters (Hands and Feet): These

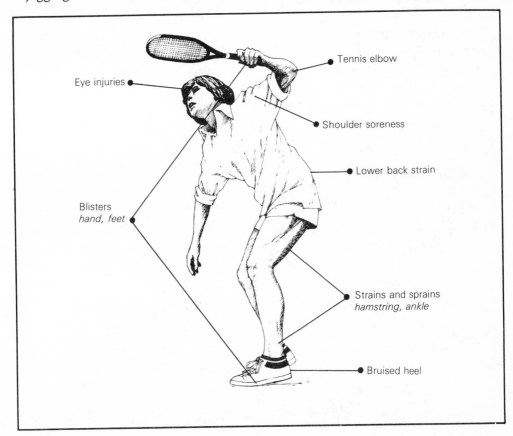

are quite common, especially at the beginning of a season. It is well worth while to harden the hands and feet with alcohol or a skin-hardening agent. Wearing gloves may be a help early in the season, but should be given up as soon as the hands are accustomed to play.

Strains and sprains: These are as frequent in racquetball as in any energetic sport involving a lot of starting and stopping and change of direction. Most vulnerable are the ankle and hamstrings. Strength and flexibility exercises during the conditioning program combined with thorough warm-up should do much to lessen or minimize these injuries.

Lower back strain: This is caused by constant stooping to retrieve a ball or by reaching to take a high ball. Flexibility and strengthening exercises for the lower back should be of help here.

Tennis elbow: This occasionally afflicts the racquetball player. For ways of easing the pain and preventing the condition, *see* Tennis, pp. 132–133.

Bruised heels: Another complaint that may afflict the racquetball player. Heel cups or padding should ease the discomfort and lessen the likelihood of recurrence.

Shoulder soreness: Usually eased by taking a hot bath or shower and flexing the shoulders while under water. This should eliminate most of the discomfort and lessen the probability of stiffness the next day.

Eye Injuries: There is a considerable risk of eye injury in racquetball, and a blow in the eye by a fast-traveling ball can be very severe. Many players now wear eye protectors or guards.

Table Tennis

TABLE TENNIS IS A SPORT that requires supreme agility. As a recreation, it demands little fitness and can be enjoyed by people of any age without prior conditioning. As a competitive sport, however, table tennis calls for considerable stamina, power, speed and a particularly high degree of mobility combined with lightning-quick reflexes and reactions.

Specific fitness for table tennis involves a high level of general conditioning allied with heart and lung endurance; flexibility in all parts of the body, especially the legs, hips, back, arms and wrists, and some strength, but not at the expense of flexibility, in the back and legs.

Alternative Sports: Swimming, cycling and running are good stamina builders. Racquet sports, especially squash and badminton, and basketball, volleyball and handball are all excellent in promoting ball control and hand/eye coordination. Gymnastics is good for general suppleness, while aikido and judo help to speed up reactions and reflexes.

Warm-Up: This usually takes the form of a little gentle jogging followed by flexibility exercises, with emphasis on the wrists and fingers.

TABLE TENNIS FITNESS EXERCISES

Flexibility

F1. Side Bends—hips and thighs
F2. Trunk Twists—trunk and neck
F3. Alternate Toe Touches—back, shoulders and arms
F7. Arm Circles—arms and upper body
F9. Wrist Shakes—wrists and hands
F11. The Lunge—groin and thigh
F14. Knee Pulls—lower leg

Strength

Strength in table tennis must not be at the expense of flexibility. Nevertheless some strengthening exercises, especially those for the back and legs, are useful.

S3. Two-Chair Push-Ups—arms and shoulders
S6. Tennis Ball Squeeze—wrists and hands

S7. Fingertip Push-Ups—fingers
S8. Fingertip Hip Raises—fingers
S9. "Bicycling"—abdomen
S11. Half Squats—thighs
S17. Bench Jumps—upper leg
S18. Shin Strengtheners—lower leg
S19. Calf Raises—lower leg

In addition, weight training under supervision: low resistance, high-repetition exercises concentrating on the back and upper legs.

Heart and Lung

Running, particularly Fartlek and interval training; shuttle runs (10–15-yard maximum), zigzags and sprints for developing speed; lateral and backward running are also good
Ropework
Swimming
Cycling

HOME CIRCUIT

Preliminary warm-up
Jogging on the spot
Ropework, if appropriate, otherwise jogging
F7. Arm Circles
S11. Half Squats
F2. Trunk Twists
S9. "Bicycling"
F11. The Lunge

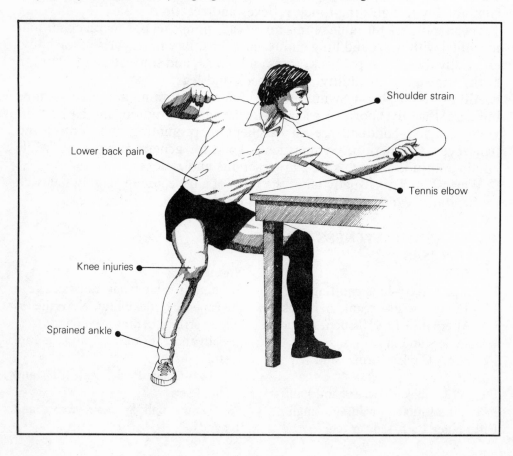

Shoulder strain

Lower back pain

Tennis elbow

Knee injuries

Sprained ankle

S17. Bench Jumps
F3. Alternate Toe Touches
S8. Fingertip Hip Raises

TABLE TENNIS INJURIES

Lower Back Strain: This is particularly prevalent due to the current use of heavy top spin and lift in playing a shot. Strength and flexibility exercises should make this less likely.

Shoulder Strain: The shoulder is aggravated by constant play. Strength and flexibility exercises should give some immunity.

Tennis Elbow: Due largely to the wristy nature of some shots. (*See* Tennis, pp. 132–133, for treatment and some preventative measures.)

Ankle Injuries: These are probably the most common table tennis injuries and are almost treated as occupational hazards by players. Ankle-strengthening and flexibility exercises should help prevent these injuries.

Knee Injuries: These vary from simple sprains to severe cartilage trouble, and are almost always caused by sudden quick twists or turns. Knee-strengthening exercises are a useful preventative.

Falls: Falling injuries vary from cuts, abrasions and bruises, severe or mild, to the very occasional fracture.

Swimming

SWIMMING IS ONE OF the most popular recreations, and as such requires little prior fitness to be thoroughly enjoyed. Competition swimming, on the other hand, is a sport that demands great stamina and specific strengths, as well as a good degree of all-around suppleness.

Specific fitness for general swimming calls for a high degree of heart and lung endurance. It requires strength in the arms, shoulders and abdomen—in addition, the back stroke requires strong legs, while the breast stroke calls for strong legs and also a strong back. Flexibility is also needed, especially in the shoulders and knees.

Alternative Sports: More swimming is far and away the best stamina builder for swimmers. Ropework is also popular as are running, walking or jogging. Squash is good for building strength and suppleness, while basketball and volleyball are good for general body coordination.

Warm-Up: This usually takes the form of some jogging followed by flexibility exercises out of the water; and then some long distance and shorter sprint swims.

SWIMMING FITNESS EXERCISES

Flexibility
F1. Side Bends—hips and thighs
F2. Trunk Twists—trunk and neck
F3. Alternate Toe Touches—back, shoulders and arms
F4. Neck Rolls—neck
F7. Arm Circles—arms and upper body
F11. The Lunge—groin and thighs
F14. Knee Pulls—lower leg
F15. Calf Stretches—lower leg

In addition, try the **Dive Loosener** (*see* Diving, p. 151).

Strength
S1. Push-Ups or Modified Push-Ups—body
S2. Pull-Ups—arms and shoulders
S3. Two-Chair Push-Ups—arms and shoulders

S10. Bent-Leg Sit-Ups—abdomen
S13. Sprinters—thighs
S16. Step-Ups—upper legs
S17. Bench Jumps—upper leg

In addition, weight training under supervision, especially for the back, arms and shoulders.

Heart and Lung
Running
Jogging on the spot
Ropework

HOME CIRCUIT
Preliminary warm-up
Jogging on the spot
Ropework, if appropriate; otherwise jogging
S1. Push-Ups or Modified Push-Ups
F2. Trunk Twists
F11. The Lunge
S16. Step-Ups
F3. Alternate Toe Touches
S10. Bent-Leg Sit-Ups

F4. Neck Rolls
S13. Sprinters
F13. Knee Pulls

SWIMMING INJURIES
The cushioning effect of the water and the fact that there is no contact with the ground eliminate a lot of "normal" sports injuries. Swimming is thus a comparatively injury-free sport, provided a proper warm-up is carried out before a swim followed by a good warm-down afterwards.

Muscle strains do occur, especially to the back and shoulder, and often as a result of overtraining. The shoulder is particularly vulnerable in the crawl and this can result in "Swimmer's Shoulder" when constant shoulder rotation can lead to sprain of the joint or irritation of the muscle. Strength and flexibility exercises in the conditioning program and a really thorough warm-up and warm-down before and after

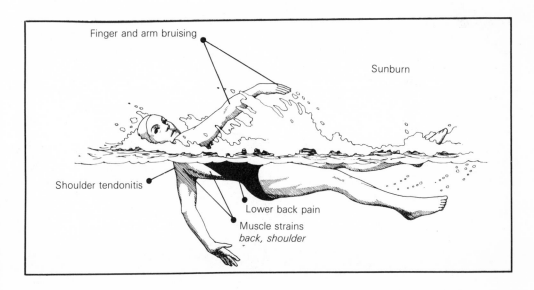

swimming should do much to minimize these injuries.

Lower back pain can also cause considerable trouble with a swimmer and could prove a major handicap unless treated professionally at the first sign. However, flexibility and strengthening exercises will help avoid this.

Tendonitis of the shoulder (particularly with back strokers) **and the knee** also occasionally occurs. Thorough conditioning and warm-up are essential in helping to avoid this, and it is also important to ensure that the shoulder does not get chilled after exertion.

Finger and arm bruising can occur on turns, from hitting the end of the pool, but this is not usually severe.

The reflecting power of water on sunlight can cause severe **sunburn** on exposed parts of the body. Until you are accustomed to the sun's rays, either wear a T-shirt or use some form of barrier cream. In very bright sun even a T-shirt gives only partial protection; so it is essential to limit one's exposure. It is impossible to lay down guidelines on this; commonsense and an awareness of the risk of sunburn in water must dictate.

Diving

DIVING REQUIRES A high standard of general fitness, explosive strength in the legs, strength in the stomach and back (to enable the diver to hold line on entry into the water) as well as in shoulders, wrists and forearms. In addition, it calls for very quick reflexes and considerable flexibility, especially in the hips, back, upper legs and calves.

Alternative Sports: Racquet sports, such as squash and badminton, and volleyball are useful alternative sports, assisting with general strengthening and suppling of the body. Running, jogging and, of course, swimming are excellent stamina builders.

Warm-Up: As with most sports, the warm-up in diving is quite essential. This usually takes the form of gentle jogging, followed by flexibility exercises.

DIVING FITNESS EXERCISES
Flexibility

F1. Side Bends—hips and thighs
F2. Trunk Twists—trunk and neck
F4. Neck Rolls—neck
F7. Arm Circles—arms and upper body
F9. Wrist Shakes—wrists and hands
F11. The Lunge—groin and thighs
F12. Hurdles—groin and thighs

In addition, the **Dive Loosener** is a good swimming and diving flexibility exercise: Stand erect, feet comfortably apart, knees slightly bent, arms hanging loosely at the sides. Bend forward until the hands almost touch the ground. Drop the head forward, relaxing the neck muscles. Swing both arms backwards and forwards, bending the knees even more on the forward movement and straightening them on the backward motion. Keep all muscles as relaxed as possible, and the movements smooth and rhythmical.

Strength

S1. Push-Ups or Modified Push-Ups
  —body
S2. Pull-Ups—arm and shoulders
S5. Broomstick Rolls—wrists and hands
S10. Bent-Leg Sit-Ups—abdomen
S11. Half Squats—thighs
S12. Squat Thrusts—thighs
S15. Leg Raises—upper leg
S16. Step-Ups—upper leg
S17. Bench Jumps—upper leg
S19. Calf Raises—lower leg

Heart and Lung

Running
Jogging
Ropework
Swimming

HOME CIRCUIT

Preliminary warm-up
Jogging on the spot
Ropework, if appropriate; otherwise jogging
S1. Push-Ups or Modified Push-Ups
S10. Bent-Leg Sit-Ups
F12. Hurdles
F2. Trunk Twists
S16. Step-Ups
F7. Arm Circles
S12. Squat Thrusts

DIVING INJURIES

As in most other sports, diving injuries are more frequent and often more serious the more tense the competitor. Skill and experience gives confidence, which the diver must have—along with requis-

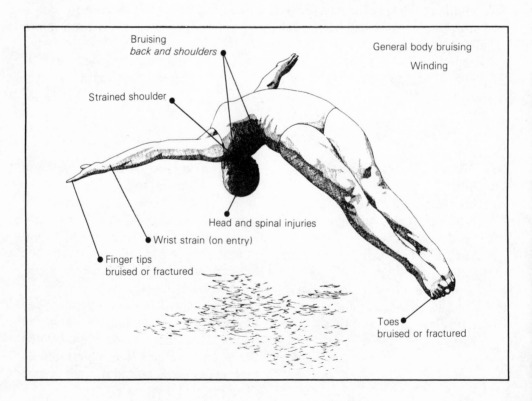

Bruising *back and shoulders*

General body bruising

Winding

Strained shoulder

Head and spinal injuries

Wrist strain (on entry)

Finger tips bruised or fractured

Toes bruised or fractured

ite physical ability—before taking on a new dive. The relaxing effect of the warm-up for a diver is in some ways just as important as the more physical benefits.

Many divers suffer from general **body bruises** caused when entering the water. For the most part, these are not severe and any discomfort usually disappears after a hot bath or shower combined with gentle flexing exercises under water. Bad entry, on the other hand, can cause more severe bruising, especially to the back and shoulders. The treatment here is application of ice. It is important to keep the shoulder mobile to prevent stiffening.

Flattening the hand to ensure a clean entry is inclined to lead to **wrist strain or wrench.** Strengthening the wrist and forearm muscles should lessen the likelihood of this.

Winding is quite frequent following a "belly flop" on entry. The victims can usually make their own way to the side of the bath where they can be helped

out. But anyone in attendance should be particularly watchful after a really bad entry. Having helped the diver on to dry land, allow him to rest for a few minutes—the feeling of breathlessness usually passes very quickly. Thereafter, reassurance is the only treatment usually needed.

Fingertips and toes may be **bruised** or occasionally **broken** after contact with the board upon take off. In addition, **shoulder muscles** may also be **strained.**

By far the most potentially serious injuries are those to **head, back or spine**; these can be fatal or cause irreparable damage. For details of water rescue, *see* Part III. It is vitally important to ensure that the head and body are kept in a straight line, otherwise the spinal column may be injured. Many pools and swimming areas provide spinal boards; others have stretchers on to which the injured person can be eased and then carefully and slowly brought on to dry land.

Sailing

SAILING AT THE recreational level can be enjoyed with little or no prior conditioning, apart from some hand hardening to prevent blisters. But racing—either small-boat racing or sail-cruise racing—requires very considerable stamina, specific strengths and a high degree of general body suppleness.

In small-boat racing, crew members need to be fitter than the helmsman, but both must be as fit as athletes. In particular, single-helm sailing calls for a very high standard of all-round fitness as it is one of the most exacting and exhausting sports there is. Small-boat racing requires very swift reflexes, excellent body coordination and balance. Small-boat sailors need a high level of heart and lung endurance; they also require strength in the thighs, abdomen and lower back (as these are placed under immense strain during trapeze work and while hanging out) and in the arms, wrists and hands (for sail handling and coping with the many emergencies that are bound to occur). In addition, all-round body flexibility is needed.

Sail cruising and sail racing require a high level of heart and lung endurance, especially for long-distance or ocean races. They also require both all-around strength and specific strength in the upper body, arms, wrists and hands—not for nothing are the crews of the big boats called "gorillas." In addition, general suppleness and agility are required, not only for sail handling but for avoiding injury in stormy weather.

Alternative Sports: For general stamina building for all types of sailing, running, jogging, cycling, swimming and ropework are all excellent. Racquet games, such as squash and badminton, are useful agility sports, especially for the small-boat sailor.

Sailors should try to keep generally fit during the off-season period. Many take to team games such as soccer or field hockey. There is now, however, a tendency for small-boat sailing to go on throughout the year in some countries.

Warm-Up: In small-boat racing this usually takes the form of some gentle jogging followed by flexibility exercises. It is important to keep the exertion well below the sweating level due to the risk of chilling during the sail. On the sail out it is usual to go through all the motions and manoeuvres that will be needed during the actual race.

SAILING FITNESS EXERCISES

Flexibility
F1. Side Bends—hips and thighs
F2. Trunk Twists—trunk and neck
F3. Alternate Toe Touches—back, shoulders and arms
F4. Neck Rolls—neck
F9. Wrist Shakes—wrists and hands
F11. The Lunge—groin and thighs
F15. Calf Stretches—lower leg

Strength
S1. Push-Ups or Modified Push-Ups —body
S2. Pull-Ups—arms and shoulders
S5. Broomstick Rolls—wrists and hands
S9. "Bicycling"—abdomen
S10. Bent-Leg Sit-Ups—abdomen
S12. Squat Thrusts—thighs

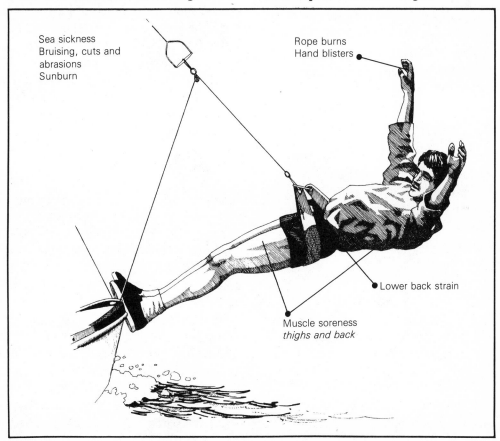

Sea sickness
Bruising, cuts and abrasions
Sunburn

Rope burns
Hand blisters

Lower back strain

Muscle soreness
thighs and back

S15. Leg Raises—upper leg

S17. Bench Jumps—upper leg

In addition, weight training under supervision, especially for the back, abdomen and upper leg.

The **Cat Dip** (*see* Judo, p. 121) is another excellent sailing exercise. It both supples and strengthens the back, and is also useful for stamina building.

Heart and Lung

Running, especially Fartlek and interval training, sprints and uphill work

Jogging

Ropework

Cycling

Swimming

HOME CIRCUIT

Preliminary warm-up

Jogging on the spot

Ropework, if appropriate; otherwise jogging

F2. Trunk Twists

S1. Push-Ups Modified Push-Ups

F3. Alternate Toe Touches

S10. Bent-Leg Sit-Ups

F4. Neck Rolls

S15. Leg Raises

S2. Pull-Ups

S12. Squat Thrusts

SAILING INJURIES

In general, most sailing injuries are due to the action of wind, weather and water, and the sailor is particularly susceptible to **bruising, cuts, abrasions** and, occasionally, **fractures.**

Rope burns and **blisters on the hand** are other occupational hazards of the sailor. Blisters and cuts should be dealt with as soon as they start to form, as the tendency is for them to become waterlogged; which in turn opens them to infection. At the start of the season many sailors wear gloves until their hands have hardened sufficiently. Anyone who is susceptible to getting blisters is advised to set about hardening the hands, either with alcohol or a skin-hardening agent, well before the sailing season starts. **Sunburn** is also very prevalent, especially to the face.

Muscle soreness, especially around the thighs and in the back, is quite common with small-boat sailors, due to the constant effort involved in hanging out. The latter activity can also lead to **lower back strain.** It is very important that preseason conditioning include a lot of work on the back, abdomen and upper leg. This, in combination with thorough stretching, should do much to lessen the likelihood of lower back trouble.

Seasickness is at best extremely unpleasant; in extreme form it can be totally incapacitating. It usually gets worse as the weather deteriorates and the water gets rougher, which is unfortunate as this is the time when the crew needs to be at their most alert. The condition is aggravated by fatigue, cold and hunger.

To counteract seasickness, general all-round fitness is very beneficial. Avoid fatty and greasy foods in the diet, and eat simple foods when on the water. Make sure that the occasional hot drink is taken, such as soup, cocoa or coffee. Various "witches remedies" are often recommended by those subject to seasickness. These vary from chewing on a dry crust of bread to chewing gum. Others suggest that seasickness is all in the mind—usually those who don't suffer from it—and therefore you should ignore it.

Seasickness pills are very effective, but some may cause drowsiness; so it is as well to try to discover the one most suited to your own case. In any event, the effects of seasickness usually wear off within 48 hours. If practical, ensure that the cabin is well ventilated; there is nothing worse than the smell of stale air, cooking odors and engine oil in the cabin of a tossing boat when you feel sick to your stomach.

Rowing

ROWING IS PHYSICALLY exacting as both a recreational pursuit and as a competitive sport. A generally relaxing and liberating activity, it is gaining wide popularity among those with ready access to water who find jogging tedious. Doctors recommend that anyone over 30 who takes up rowing or sculling for the first time, or picks it up again after a long lay-off, should have a thorough medical examination.

Specifically, rowing requires a high degree of heart and lung endurance; strength, particularly in the trunk and back, neck, abdomen and legs; and flexibility in the back, body, hips, arms, wrists, knees, ankles and heels.

Alternative Sports: Running, jogging, swimming and cycling are alternative stamina builders, but nothing can really substitute for rowing itself. Racquet sports, particularly squash and badminton, as well as basketball and volleyball are useful as they require (and promote) a high degree of back flexibility.

Warm-Up: Jogging and flexibility exercises on land; on the water some gentle rowing interspersed with short rowing sprints should gradually prepare the muscles for extended use. Tracksuit tops or sweaters, etc., should be worn to the last moment, especially in cold weather.

ROWING FITNESS EXERCISES
Flexibility
F1. Side Bends—hips and thighs
F2. Trunk Twists—trunk and neck
F3. Alternate Toe Touches—back, shoulders and arms
F6. Wing Stretchers—shoulders
F10. The Reach—stomach, thigh and calves
F12. Hurdles—groin and thigh
F14. Knee Pulls—lower leg
F15. Calf Stretches—lower leg

Strength
S1. Push-Ups or Modified Push-Ups —body
S2. Pull-Ups—arms and shoulders
S10. Bent-Leg Sit-Ups—abdomen
S11. Half Squats—thighs

S12. Squat Thrusts—thighs
S16. Step-Ups—upper leg
S17. Bench Jumps—upper leg

In addition, weight training under supervision.

Heart and Lung
Rowing
Running, especially cross-country
Jogging
Swimming
Cycling

HOME CIRCUIT
Ropework, if appropriate; otherwise jogging
S1. Push-Ups or Modified Push-Ups
F2. Trunk Twists
F12. Hurdles
S10. Bent-Leg Sit-Ups

F3. Alternate Toe Touches
S2. Pull-Ups
S16. Step-Ups
S12. Squat Thrust

ROWING INJURIES
Many rowing injuries can be avoided with proper strengthening and flexibility exercises in conjunction with a thorough warm-up before taking to the water.

Blisters (Hands): These are most common at the beginning of the season, before the hands have had a chance to harden up. They are also caused by gripping the oar too tight. (This tendency, particularly in beginners, can also lead to **tenosynovitis of the wrist**). It is well worth hardening the hands before the beginning of the rowing

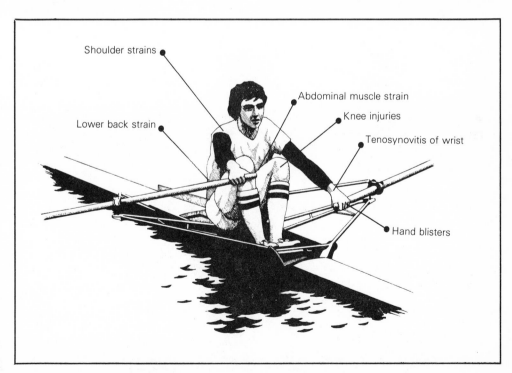

Shoulder strains

Lower back strain

Abdominal muscle strain

Knee injuries

Tenosynovitis of wrist

Hand blisters

season either with alcohol or some skin-hardening agent.

Lower Back (also Shoulder) Strain: This is sometimes caused during rowing training, particularly in lifting a weight awkwardly; however it is more frequently due to incorrect technique. If chronic or recurring, it is worth consulting a coach.

Abdominal Muscle Strain: This usually occurs at the start of the season and is due to inadequate strengthening and stretching exercises and/or warm-up.

Knee Injuries: Usually to the knee-cap and occurs during the drive off the stretcher. An imbalance between the quadriceps muscles at the front of the thigh and the hamstrings at the back is usually the cause. This can be remedied by balanced exercises for the two muscle groups.

Canoeing

CANOEING IS A WIDELY popular sport in both its single-paddle form (canoe) and its double-paddle form (kayak). Both varieties require a degree of stamina, whether at the recreational or competitive level. Canoeing is looked upon as an excellent stamina builder, and many people find it both exhilarating and relaxing as an exercise.

Specifically, **canoeing** at the competitive level requires a high degree of heart and lung endurance; strength in the back, shoulders, arms and legs; and flexibility in the hips as well as the shoulders and wrists. **Kayaking** requires a high degree of heart and lung endurance; strength in the back, shoulders and arms; and flexibility in the lower back, shoulders, wrists and upper leg.

Alternative Sports: In general canoeists choose alternative or off-season sports that have a low risk of injury. For canoe, skiing, especially Nordic skiing, is popular; for kayak, racquet games, swimming and field events such as the shot put or hammer throw are favorites. For both forms of canoeing, running, jogging and cycling are excellent stamina builders.

Warm-Up: The warm-up before canoeing is very important and usually comprises a gentle jog on land, followed by flexibility exercises, with particular emphasis on the back and shoulders and, for canoe, the hips as well.

CANOEING FITNESS EXERCISES

Flexibility

F1. Side Bends—hips and thighs
F2. Trunk Twists—trunk and neck
F3. Alternate Toe Touches—back, shoulders and arms
F4. Neck Rolls—neck
F6. Wing Stretchers—shoulders
F7. Arm Circles—arms and upper body
F9. Wrist Shakes—wrists and hands
F12. Hurdles—groin and thigh
F13. Leg Swings—upper body

Strength

S1. Push-Ups or Modified Push-Ups
—body

S2. Pull-Ups—arms and shoulders

S3. Two-Chair Push-Ups—arms and shoulders

S5. Broomstick Rolls—wrists and hands

S6. Tennis Ball Squeeze—wrists and hands

S10. Bent-Leg Sit-Ups—abdomen

S12. Squat Thrusts—thighs

S16. Step-Ups—upper leg

In addition, weight training under supervision, especially for back, shoulders, arms and legs.

Heart and Lung

Running, especially Fartlek and interval training

Jogging

Cycling

Ropework

HOME CIRCUIT

Preliminary warm-up

Ropework, if appropriate; otherwise jogging

S1. Push-Ups or Modified Push-Ups

F2. Trunk Twists

S10. Bent-Leg Sit-Ups

S2. Pull-Ups

F4. Neck Rolls

F7. Arm Circles

S3. Two-Chair Push-Ups

S12. Squat Thrusts

CANOEING INJURIES

Many canoeing injuries, especially strains and sprains, are due either to incorrect technique or inadequate warm-up. Tension in the inexperienced is also a major contributory factor (to muscle strain in particular).

Blisters: Especially on the hand at the start of the season. For the kayak canoeist these often occur on the inside

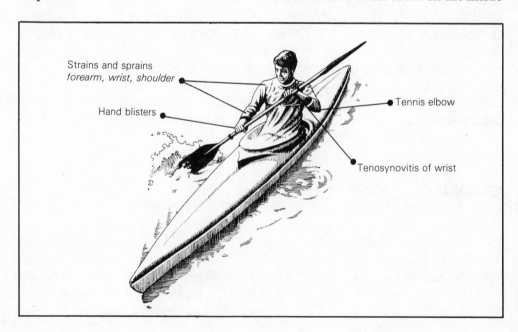

of the thumb. It is essential to carry out hand-hardening using alcohol or a skin-hardening agent before setting about canoeing in earnest.

Tennis Elbow: This is a quite common ailment among canoeists. For treatment and ways of easing the discomfort, *see* Tennis, pp. 132–133. Rest is the only long-term solution.

Strains and Sprains: Usually to the forearms, wrists or shoulders. In extreme cases of shoulder strain, bursitis may also develop. **Tenosynovitis** also occurs to the wrist in canoeing, probably due to gripping the paddle too tightly and not letting the wrist relax sufficiently. Flexibility and strength exercises and a really thorough warm-up before taking to the water should do much to lessen the incidence of these injuries.

Surfing

SURFING IS A SPORT that requires the participant to be, above all, a confident and competent swimmer. It is a very exacting sport and liable to tax the unfit to the limit of their endurance. It calls for agility, balance, suppleness, timing and a sense of rhythm.

Specific fitness for surfing demands a high standard of general fitness and heart and lung endurance; strength, especially in the upper body, legs and calves; and all-around flexibility.

Alternative Sports: Swimming, especially the crawl, is the ideal way for the surfer to gain heart and lung endurance. Running, jogging and cycling are also good. Gymnastics and free-style skating both encourage similar degrees of mobility, and yoga is excellent for general relaxation.

Warm-Up: Jogging, followed by flexibility exercises, especially for the back and legs.

SURFING FITNESS EXERCISES

Flexibility

F1. Side Bends—hips and thighs
F2. Trunk Twists—trunk and neck
F3. Alternate Toe Touches—back, shoulders and arms
F4. Neck Rolls—neck
F7. Arm Circles—arms and upper body
F10. The Reach—stomach, thighs and calves
F12. Hurdles—groin and thighs
F14. Knee Pulls—lower legs

Strength

S1. Push-Ups or Modified Push-Ups —body
S2. Pull-Ups—arms and shoulders
S9. "Bicycling"—abdomen
S10. Bent-Leg Sit-Ups—abdomen
S12. Squat Thrusts—thighs (an excellent surfing exercise)
S16. Step-Ups—upper leg
S19. Calf Raises—lower leg

In addition, weight training under supervision, especially for the upper body and legs.

Heart and Lung
Swimming, especially the crawl
Running, especially Fartlek and interval training
Cycling
Ropework

In addition, deep breathing exercises designed to develop and strengthen the surfer's ability to hold breath underwater are invaluable.

HOME CIRCUIT
Ropework, if appropriate; otherwise jogging.
S1. Push-Ups or Modified Push-Ups
F2. Trunk Twists
F12. Hurdles
S10. Bent-Leg Sit-Ups
F4. Neck Rolls
S16. Step-Ups
F3. Alternate Toe Touches
S19. Calf Raises
S16. Squat Thrusts

SURFING INJURIES
Surfing is relatively free from major injury, unless surfers run into one another or are too inexperienced to cope with large waves. It is essential that every surfer is fully aware of other surfers and swimmers nearby. A surfboard particularly in the hands of a novice can be a lethal projectile.

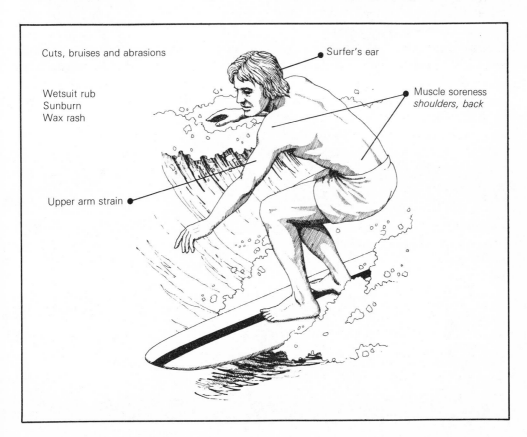

Cuts, bruises and abrasions

Wetsuit rub
Sunburn
Wax rash

Surfer's ear

Muscle soreness
shoulders, back

Upper arm strain

Cuts, Bruises and Abrasions: These do occur, but more often out of the water than in, unless a collision takes place (this is particularly common with new and inexperienced surfers). Damaged boards, or those which haven't been repaired properly, often have sharp edges or splinters of fiberglass which can cause injury. In very warm climates cuts and wounds should be treated immediately.

Arm Strain: Particularly in the muscles of the upper arm. This happens from time to time as a result of a long paddle out. Flexibility and strengthening exercises combined with a thorough warm-up before entering the water should do much to avoid this injury.

Muscle soreness is common, particularly with new surfers. This is usually felt in the lower back and shoulders and is often the result of tension and/or a wrong distribution of weight while surfing. Taking a hot bath or shower and flexing the muscles while under water should minimize the discomfort and prevent stiffness the next day.

Wet suit rub is particularly common on arms and shoulders. Many surfers use vaseline or some form of gel to lubricate the sore area and reduce friction between the skin and the wet suit rubber. However, constant application of vaseline can cause rubber to rot.

Sunburn can be vicious in surfing. The bridge of the nose is particularly vulnerable. Zinc oxide ointment acts as a very good barrier cream. The upper body can also get badly burned and, until they are used to the sun, many surfers, especially at the start of the season, wear T-shirts.

T-shirts can also prevent **wax rash**, which is caused by lying on the board.

Surfer's ear is a common condition that over the years may gradually impair the hearing. It is caused by cold breeze or wind continually rushing past the ear and results in a boney growth gradually developing in the ear canal. Wearing ear plugs or a wet suit hood are satisfactory preventatives.

Windsurfing

WINDSURFING IS AN EXCELLENT all-around form of exercise that requires technique, experience and balance, rather than any excessive degree of strength or agility. It does not call for great powers of endurance; but the fitter the windsurfer the better, especially when contending with strong winds and a choppy sea. Recreational windsurfing has an advantage over conventional sailing in that the surfer can stop when tired by dropping the sail in the water and when rested take up the boom again and continue.

A relatively new sport, windsurfing is becoming increasingly competitive and, as such, is turning into a highly physical sport. Windsurf racing—which takes the form of slalom-style, free-style or long-distance events (up to 15 miles)—demands considerable stamina, strength and agility. Buoyball (another form of windsurfing akin to a kind of rugby on water) calls for an extremely high level of fitness.

Specific fitness for windsurfing involves a degree of heart and lung endurance; strength in the upper body (especially at first, when the newcomer to the sport is very tense) and more particularly in the back, arms and legs; and flexibility in hips, shoulders, and upper and lower legs.

Alternative Sports: Racquet sports, especially squash and badminton, are useful off-season activities. Running, swimming and cycling are good stamina builders. Snow skiing and water skiing, with their emphasis on balance, are excellent conditioners for windsurfing. Surfing improves balance, while dinghy sailing can help the windsurfer develop a feel for the wind.

Warm-Up: The warm-up is important in both recreational and competitive windsurfing, because physical effort begins as soon as the surfer hoists the sail. Carry out a little gentle jogging and some flexibility exercises.

WINDSURFING FITNESS
EXERCISES
Flexibility
F1. Side Bends—hips and thighs

F2. Trunk Twists—trunk and neck

F3. Alternative Toe Touches—back, shoulders and arms

F7. Arm Circles—arms and upper body

F12. Hurdles—groin and thigh

F14. Knee Pulls—lower leg

An excellent exercise for windsurfers to improve their balance is **Ball and Board**. This consists of balancing on a board (3 feet long and 1 foot wide is ideal) to the underneath of which has been nailed a solid rubber or wooden ball. (The ball should be nailed to the centre of the board).

Strength
S1. Push-Ups or Modified Push-Ups —body

S2. Pull-Ups—arms and shoulders

S5. Broomstick Rolls—wrists and hands

S6. Tennis Ball Squeeze—wrists and hands

S10. Bent-Leg Sit-Ups—abdomen

S11. Half Squats—thighs (*particularly important as windsurfing is mainly carried out in a half-squat position*)

S12. Squat Thrusts—thighs

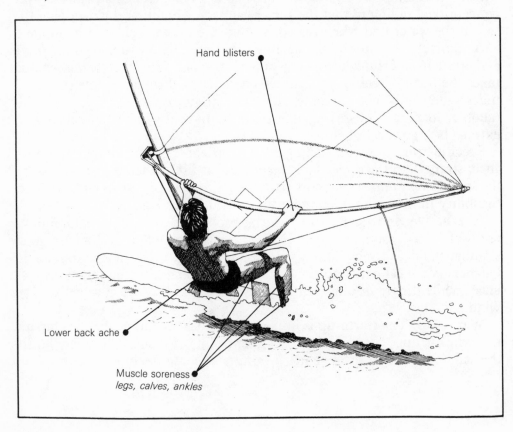

Hand blisters

Lower back ache

Muscle soreness
legs, calves, ankles

The **Wall Sit** (Phantom Chair), *see* Skiing p. 181, is another very useful windsurfing exercise.

Heart and Lung
Running
Jogging
Swimming

HOME CIRCUIT
Preliminary warm-up
Jogging on the spot
Ropework, if appropriate; otherwise jogging
S1. Push-Ups or Modified Push-Ups
F2. Trunk Twists
S2. Pull-Ups
F12. Hurdles
S10. Bent-Leg Sit-Ups
F3. Alternate Toe Touches
Wall Sits (*see* Skiing, p. 181)
F14. Knee Pulls

WINDSURFING INJURIES
Windsurfing is an almost injury-free sport. Novices in particular, however, are prone to **muscle soreness** in the legs, calves and ankles. This is caused by poor technique combined with tension. As technique and experience improve, the tendency to develop muscle soreness usually disappears.

Blisters may occur initially until the hands are hardened. Applications of alcohol or a skin-hardening agent will speed the hardening process.

Lower back ache is the most common complaint. It is due to the almost permanent semi-crouched stance of the windsurfer. A hot bath or shower and gentle flexing under water usually soothes the ache. The condition tends to be aggravated by tension and soon disappears as the windsurfer develops better technique and confidence.

Water accidents are rare in windsurfing as the surfer has a guaranteed permanently floating board to swim to should he or she fall off (this is because the board stops dead as soon as the sail falls in the water). The sport is considered so safe that life jackets are not required and lifeguards are increasingly using windsurfing boards as rescue craft.

Water Skiing

WATER SKIING IS A SPORT that, although it does not require great stamina, does demand intense and concentrated physical effort for short periods of time.

Specifically, water skiing requires a high standard of general fitness; strength, particularly in the upper and lower trunk, arms, wrists and legs, and flexibility in hips, shoulders, wrists and legs.

Alternative Sports: Squash, badminton, gymnastics and trampoline work are all beneficial to the water skier as alternative or off-season sports. Snow skiing, both Nordic and alpine, is the most nearly approximate alternative sport and many water skiers are as proficient on the snow as they are on the water. Running, cycling and swimming are useful stamina builders.

Warm-Up: Most water skiing injuries are associated with or heightened by tension, so warming-up before taking to the water is essential. This usually takes the form of some gentle jogging followed by flexibility exercises, with emphasis on hips, shoulders, arms and legs.

WATER SKIING EXERCISES
Flexibility
F1. Side Bends—hips and thighs
F2. Trunk Twists—trunk and neck
F3. Alternate Toe Touches—back, shoulders and arms
F4. Neck Rolls—neck
F7. Arm Circles—arms and upper body
F9. Wrist Shakes—wrists and hands
F11. The Lunge—groin and thighs
F14. Knee Pulls—lower legs

Strength
S1. Push-Ups or Modified Push-Ups —body
S2. Pull-Ups—arms and shoulders
S3. Two-Chair Push-Ups—arms and shoulders
S5. Broomstick Rolls—wrists and hands
S10. Bent-Leg Sit-Ups—abdomen
S12. Squat Thrusts—thighs
S16. Step-Ups—upper leg
S19. Calf Raises—lower leg

In addition, weight training under supervision, usually in the off-season period and with emphasis on upper and lower trunk, arms and legs.

Heart and Lung
Running, particularly Fartlek and interval training
Jogging
Cycling
Swimming
Ropework

HOME CIRCUIT
Preliminary warm-up
Ropework, if appropriate; otherwise jogging
S1. Push-Ups
F2. Trunk Twists
F11. The Lunge
S10. Bent-Leg Sit-Ups
S16. Step-Ups
F7. Arm Circles
S3. Two-Chair Push-Ups
S12. Squat Thrusts

WATER SKIING INJURIES
There is a vastly increased risk of injury in water skiing when the skier is suffering from tension. It is important therefore for the skier to quickly build up confidence in his or her own skill and ability. The importance of the warm-up cannot be overstressed.

Cuts, Abrasions and Rope Burns: These can all be caused when the skier falls into the water and the rope winds round or lashes out. Frequently the arms and legs are injured in this way.

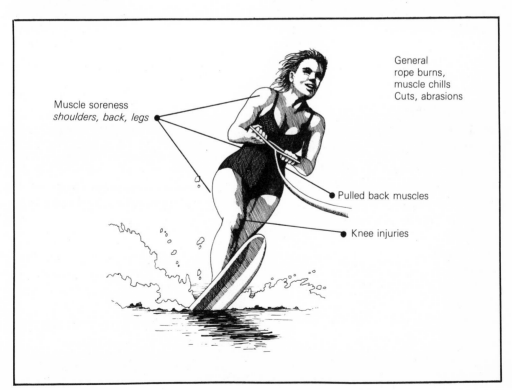

Muscle soreness *shoulders, back, legs*

General rope burns, muscle chills Cuts, abrasions

Pulled back muscles

Knee injuries

Muscle soreness: Beginners are particularly vulnerable to general muscle soreness. A hot bath will get rid of most of the discomfort.

Back injuries: Particularly to the lower back, and mainly pulled muscles. A high standard of general fitness and conditioning aimed at strengthening the back muscles, together with thorough warming-up before skiing, should do much to prevent these injuries.

Knee injuries: Usually ligament or muscle pulls, occasionally cartilage trouble. A strengthening and flexibility regime before and during the skiing season should help prevent these.

Clothing: Water skiing is a far colder sport than it appears, on any but the hottest days it is best to wear some form of jersey or sweater to avoid muscle chills.

Water Polo

WATER POLO IS AN exacting sport requiring a high standard of general fitness. (Anyone taking it up for the first time, unless already reasonably fit, should have a medical checkup beforehand.)

Swimming endurance is the first need. With 5 minutes of actual playing time allowed in each of the 4 quarters (which means, due to various delays, in reality nearer 10 minutes) the player will be either swimming or treading water for a considerable period. Within that time, short bursts of swimming speed are required, also explosive uses of the muscles in "lifting" the body out of the water for passing, intercepting or shooting. In addition, the necessary man-to-man marking and the contact nature of the game is extremely exhausting.

Specifically, in addition to swimming endurance and speed, water polo requires strength in the body, arms and legs; and flexibility in the upper body, arms, legs and ankles.

Alternative Sports: Squash, tennis, volleyball, basketball, rugby, soccer and cross-country running are all useful alternative sports for the water polo player. But nothing can compare with swimming and, more particularly, more water polo, for achieving and maintaining water polo fitness.

Warm-Up: The warm-up is as important in water polo as it is in other sports requiring explosive bursts of muscle power. This usually takes the form of gentle jogging followed by flexibility exercises on land, then passing, shooting and receiving passes in the water before the game.

WATER POLO FITNESS EXERCISES

Flexibility

F2. Trunk Twists—trunk and neck

F3. Alternate Toe Touches—back, shoulders and arms

F4. Neck Rolls—neck

F7. Arm Circles—arms and upper body

F11. The Lunge—groin and thighs

F13. Leg Swings—upper legs

F14. Knee Pulls—lower legs

Strength

S1. Push-Ups—body

S2. Pull-Ups—arms and shoulders

S3. Two-Chair Push-Ups—arms and shoulders

S5. Broomstick Rolls—wrists and hands

S8. Fingertip Hip Raises—fingers

S10. Bent-Leg Sit-Ups—abdomen

S12. Squat Thrusts—thighs

S16. Step-Ups—upper leg

In addition, weight training under supervision, especially for trunk, abdomen, legs, shoulders and wrists.

Heart and Lung

On land:

Running, including Fartlek and interval training

Walking

Cycling

Ropework

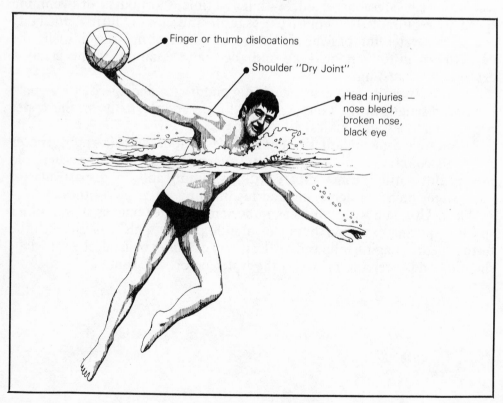

Finger or thumb dislocations

Shoulder "Dry Joint"

Head injuries — nose bleed, broken nose, black eye

On water:
Distance swimming
Fartlek and interval training (as on land)
Treading water exercises
Zigzag swimming (as on land)

HOME CIRCUIT
Preliminary warm-up
Ropework, if appropriate; otherwise jogging
S1. Push-Ups
F2. Trunk Twists
S3. Two-Chair Push-Ups
F11. The Lunge
S10. Bent-Leg Sit-Ups
S16. Step-Ups
S12. Squat Thrusts

WATER POLO INJURIES
Despite the fact that water polo appears to be a very vigorous game in which contact with opponents is frequent, water polo injuries are usually neither extensive nor severe. This is, in part, because there is no contact with the ground, and hence no solid resistance to be met by the muscles. Muscle pulls and strains are thus infrequent.

Head injuries, ranging from nose bleeds and black eyes to broken noses are quite common. **General bruising,** particularly of the upper and lower trunk, arms and legs is also quite frequent, as are **cuts and abrasions,** especially of the arms, elbows and legs. A **finger or thumb** may also suffer **dislocation** either due to a player's failing to catch the ball cleanly, or coming in contact with another player.

"Dry joint" of the shoulder is an overuse condition quite common among water polo players. It is marked by a nagging, rather than acute, pain that refuses to go away, except after total rest—which most players are reluctant to offer. It tends to recur, in any case, once play resumes.

There seems to be no permanent treatment for this condition. Strength and flexibility exercises for the shoulder help to prevent it, and treatment with ice gives local temporary relief. Most players learn to live with the condition and consider it an occupational hazard of the game. A physiotherapist should be consulted on first sign of the condition.

Underwater Swimming

SNORKEL AND SCUBA

UNDERWATER SWIMMING IS A SPORT of growing popularity and, although it can be strenuous, it calls for few specific physical requirements except an ability to swim and a reasonable level of heart and lung endurance.

Snorkeling requires swimming ability, as well as a reasonable level of heart and lung endurance; otherwise there are no specific fitness requirements.

Scuba, on the other hand, requires very considerable heart and lung endurance as well as swimming ability. Scuba swimming proficiency tests incorporate a number of mandatory skills which a would-be scuba diver must have before being allowed to start training:

- Swimming on the surface for 585 feet without stopping.
- Swimming underwater for 33 feet.
- Treading water for 3 minutes with the hands above the surface. Treading for 1 minute with hands below the surface.
- Floating on the back for 1 minute floating on the front for as long as you can.
- Jumping feet first into the deep end of a pool (8 feet) and holding the nose; then when underwater slowly blowing the air out of your lungs (a process known as equalizing) as you sink to the bottom.
- Diving head first into deep water.
- Picking up a 5-pound weight from the bottom (8 feet).

GENERAL UNDERWATER SWIMMING INJURIES

Cuts and Abrasions: These are quite common in underwater swimming, and are usually caused by sharp rocks or coral. Wounds should be treated as soon as possible, as risk of infection is high due to the likelihood of the skin around the wound becoming soggy, leaving the cut open. Be sure that the cut is thoroughly cleansed before putting on a bandage or covering.

Stings: Certain types of jelly-fish (including the Portuguese man of war) have very painful stings. If you are stung, remove the stinging trailer or tentacle-like strand using a handful of wet sand or a towel. Apply ammonia as soon as possible, followed by an anti-septic cream.

Some kinds of coral can also cause painful **blisters**. The pain from these can be relieved by applying a weak solution of ammonia followed by antiseptic cream.

Sea Urchins: Treading on a sea urchin can be extremely painful and unpleasant if the barbed spines pierce the foot. These must all be removed using tweezers. It may first be necessary to try to soften the spines: dab them with ammonia, lemon juice or some beef tenderizer, if available.

Exhaustion: This is quite a common condition and can occur without the underwater swimmer being aware of increasing fatigue or of the fact that anything at all is amiss. Exhaustion is brought on by a number of factors including:

- Continual diving, especially in cold water which is very draining on the system;

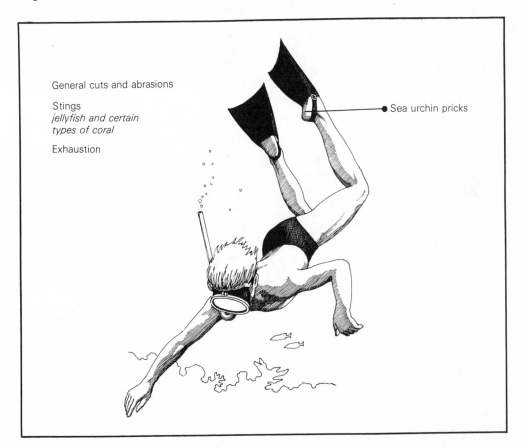

General cuts and abrasions

Stings
jellyfish and certain types of coral

Exhaustion

Sea urchin pricks

- Initial tiredness, which did not make itself felt until after diving had begun;
- Inadequate general fitness;
- General fatigue.

The onset of exhaustion can be very sudden. Sometimes, however, there is warning through a general feeling of listlessness. If this happens, get out of the water without delay. Also, *always* wear a life jacket when diving, and do not let your partner or companion get too far away—this is as much to their advantage as to yours.

General precautions:

- Never snorkel or dive without a companion.
- Find out about tides and currents before you enter the water.
- Don't be too adventurous until you know the coast or piece of water in which you are diving. This is especially important for the novice underwater swimmer.
- Keep your equipment properly maintained—your life may depend on it.

SCUBA DIVING INJURIES AND CONDITIONS

Scuba injuries and conditions nearly all derive from the effects of diving depth on the human body. (These are usually taught as an essential part of the novice scuba diver's training, and so are not covered here. The most important conditions which the divers will be instructed about are: **air embolism,** the **"bends" or decompression sickness (DCS), oxygen poisoning, nitrogen narcosis, and anoxia**). **Hypothermia** (*see* Part III) is also a complaint suffered by scuba divers.

Here are a few sensible precautions about scuba diving:

- Never dive alone.
- Never dive until you have achieved certification by a qualified club or instructor.
- Fully understand the risks, restraints and disciplines that your sport demands.
- Never dive if you are tired.
- Beware of sunstroke or seasickness on the boat journey to the diving area. Wait until these symptoms have passed before diving.
- Do not dive if you have a cold, ear or nose trouble, a heart condition or a recent operation.

Skiing

ALPINE AND NORDIC

SKIING, both alpine (downhill or slalom) and Nordic (cross-country, langlauf or ski wandering) requires stamina, strength, suppleness, good coordination and balance. The two types of skiing vary in detailed fitness requirements, but, as in all sports, fitness makes injury far less likely.

Alpine skiing is a sport which alternates between comparatively brief bursts of strenuous activity interspersed with longer periods of rest—on ski or chair lifts, or at the bottom of the slopes. The Nordic skier, on the other hand—like the cross country runner—must be able to take part in continuous activity over long periods of time.

Skiing in general, especially at high altitudes, requires endurance; strength, especially in the legs, ankles, thighs and back; and flexibility in the legs—(particularly the knees and ankles), back, hips, shoulders and arms.

Alpine skiing demands a high standard of general fitness; muscular rather than heart and lung endurance is required for the necessary brief bursts of power from legs, abdomen and upper body. Downhill skiing also requires muscular strength in the abdomen, upper trunk and upper leg muscles.

Nordic skiing essentially requires a very high level of heart and lung endurance. Leg strength, particularly in the calf muscles, is also important, as is muscle endurance in shoulders and trunk. Flexibility is called for in the waist, shoulders, upper arm (particularly the triceps) and legs.

Alternate Sports: Racquet sports, such as squash and badminton, are excellent off-season sports, as are soccer, basketball and volleyball. Swimming, cycling and running are useful stamina builders. Water skiing is the nearest summer sport to snow skiing.

Warm-Up: Warming up in skiing is doubly important, as the outside temperature is certain to be low. "Cold" muscles are especially susceptible to pulls, and to ski with "cold" muscles is an open invitation to muscle injuries. It is of little use warming up inside or outside your hotel, lodge or chalet, then waiting for a ski lift and enduring a cold ride to the top of the piste, all of which allows your body to cool down again. It is worth doing some flexibility exercises at the bottom of the piste, but reserve your greatest warm-up effort for when you arrive at the top. Here carry out gentle jogging followed by flexibility exercises—but not to the point of over sweating.

Warming-up execises (see Part I) are well worth doing at any spare moment, morning or evening. If your skiing is restricted to a few weeks in the year, start work on these at least two months before you arrive on the slopes.

ALPINE SKIING FITNESS EXERCISES

Skiing is a peculiar sport, in that some people who live far away from skiing facilities may only ski for a few weeks in the year. Many people waste valuable skiing time by not being ski-fit. Lack of fitness on the slopes is an open invitation to ski injuries, for not until fully ski-fit can the skier contend with the unexpected situations that frequently arise.

Skiing is a sport that tends to shorten the muscles of the back and the hamstrings, hence it is important that any skiing exercise routine or program include strengthening and flexibility movements for these parts of the body.

One of the best ways to attain ski fitness is using dry ski slopes, which are becoming increasingly popular.

Flexibility
F1. Side Bends—hips and thighs
F3. Alternate Toe Touches—back, shoulders and arms
F4. Neck Rolls—neck
F7. Arm Circles—arms and upper body
F9. Wrist Shakes—wrists and hands
F11. The Lunge—groin and thighs
F12. Hurdles—groin and thighs

F15. Calf Stretches—lower legs

Other useful skiing flexibility exercises are:

Off Skis
Marble Pick-Up: Sit on a chair, spread some marbles within reach on the floor, then pick them up one by one with the bare toes. This is an excellent exercise for flexing the feet and ankles.

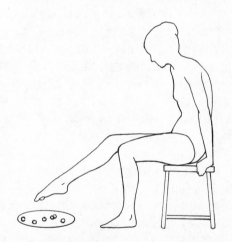

Sole Bends: When sitting on a chair, take off your shoes and bend the feet back under you so that the soles are pointing upward. Push the upper side of the ankles down toward the floor. Hold for 8 seconds, relax, then repeat. This flexes the ankle joint.

On Skis

Ski Knee Pulls: With skis on, raise one knee as high as you can, trying to keep the ski tip on the ground. Clasp the hands around the shin and pull the knee up toward the chest. Hold for 5 seconds, then return ski to the ground and repeat with the other leg. This stretches the knee, ankle, calf and foot muscles; it also is an excellent exercise for improving the balance.

Strength

S1. Push-Ups or Modified Push-Ups —body

S2. Pull-Ups—arms and shoulders

S3. Two-Chair Push-Ups—arms and shoulders

S5. Broomstick Rolls—wrists, hands

S10. Bent-Leg Sit-Ups—abdomen

S11. Half Squats—thighs

S12. Squat Thrusts—thighs

S15. Leg Raises—upper legs

S17. Bench Jumps—upper legs (also good for improving balance)

In addition, weight training under supervision, especially for the back, legs, wrists and arms.

The Wall Sit (or Phantom Chair) is an excellent exercise for strengthening the upper leg. With knees bent and back erect, lean against a wall as though a chair was there. Hold "sitting" position for as long as you can, then relax and repeat.

Heart and Lung

Running, especially Fartlek and interval training, and uphill or sandhill running. Running over rough ground also helps improve eye/foot coordination. Some skiers try slalom running through trees to help speed up their reactions. In both cases using ski sticks aids balance, as well as strengthens arms and shoulders.

Jogging

Ropework, especially skipping from a crouching position for the super-fit

Stair climbing

Swimming

Cycling

Balance

As balance is so important in skiing, a number of exercises for improving balance have been devised for the skier.

Leg Stand: This is an exercise that can be done at any time). Stand on one leg, rise on to the toes and hold for as long as you can. (This will be for a very short time at first.) Relax and repeat.

Knee Balance: Stand on one leg, raise heel off the ground and, while standing on the toes, sink down some 12 inches by bending the knee. Hold for 10 seconds then return to the upright position, repeat with the other leg.

SPECIAL FITNESS EXERCISES FOR NORDIC SKIERS

A number of alternative sports and activities are peculiarly suitable for Nordic skiers. These include all racquet games, soccer and swimming; certain track and field athletic events such as the long jump, triple jump, shot put and hurdling; and running and long walks over rough ground.

Flexibility

As for alpine skiing, with the emphasis

on the lower limbs and stride improvement, especially The Lunge (F11) and Hurdles (F12).

Strength

As for alpine skiing, but in addition all the alternatives for Push-Ups (*see* Part 1).

Roller Skis are excellent also for stamina building and to get the rhythm of the skiing movement.

Inner-Tube Stretching, using a tree or convenient post, is also a popular exercise.

Heart and Lung

Cross-country running and Fartlek and interval training are excellent for building stamina for the Nordic skier. Ropework is also popular.

HOME CIRCUIT
(for both alpine and Nordic skiers)
Preliminary warm-up
Jogging on the spot
Ropework, if appropriate; otherwise jogging
F1. Side Bends
S1. Push-Ups or Modified Push-Ups
F11. The Lunge
F3. Alternate Toe Touches
S10. Bent-Leg Sit-Ups
F7. Arm Circles
S17. Bench Jumps

In addition, the following purely skiing exercises might be attempted:

Knee Twist: Stand erect, feet together. With body upright, bend knees to 60 degrees and twist to right.

Stand up and repeat, but bending knees to left. Repeat 5 or 6 times.

Bottle Stoop: Stand erect, feet together. Place a bottle—the taller the better to start with—beside your right foot. Bend down and pick up the bottle with the *left* hand, keeping the body as upright as possible. Stand up. Place bottle by left side and pick up with right hand. Repeat 5 times each side.

Jump Twist: Stand erect, feet together. Bend knees and then jump in air, turning 90 degrees before landing on the feet. Jump again and land facing front. Repeat on the other side.

SKIING INJURIES

Skiing is a very injury-prone sport, but many skiers are unaware that many of these injuries can be prevented by sensible precautions: by using correct techniques and acquiring skiing skill; by using correct and properly maintained equipment that has been fitted by an expert; and, above all, by being fit.

Skiing injuries occur far more commonly with young or inexperienced or unfit skiers (injuries are much reduced when the novice skier is under ski instruction). Women skiers are also more prone to injury than men. In addition, fatigued athletes are always more likely to sustain injury than fit ones. In skiing this leads to an inability to cope with or react quickly enough to the unexpected. Tension, especially in the inexperienced, is also a major contributory factor to ski injuries—and tension slackens as skill and confidence grow. Tension also has a cumulative effect on shoulder soreness—due to holding an awkward position and gripping the ski poles too tightly.

General Equipment Maintenance —The Ski Boot: The ski boot must match the anatomy of the skier's leg. Ski boots provide the connection between the skier and the ski on the ground, so they must be soft enough and comfortable enough to absorb the jarring effect of skiing on rough- or hard-packed snow. The rigid link between boot and ski is provided by the ski bindings. Not only must the boots be compatible with the bindings, but the bindings themselves must be so adjusted that the boot will separate from the ski before enough force is exerted on the skier's leg to cause injury. Improperly adjusted or jamming bindings will not separate in time.

Binding Care: Ski bindings should be covered when skis are being transported on the roof of a car or when left outside in order to prevent snow or ice packing in the mechanism. Salt spray from road gritting has an appalling effect on ski bindings. Freezing of bindings can also occur if there is a wide fluctuation of temperature—as possibly in a hot room and at the top of ski-lift.

To ensure bindings are working properly, open and close them several times before finally fastening them over

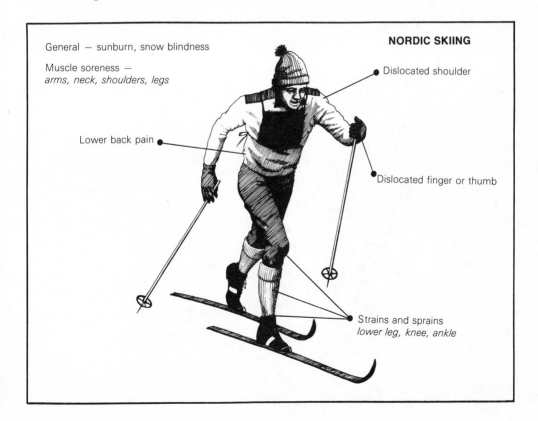

General — sunburn, snow blindness

Muscle soreness —
arms, neck, shoulders, legs

Lower back pain

NORDIC SKIING

Dislocated shoulder

Dislocated finger or thumb

Strains and sprains
lower leg, knee, ankle

the boots. They must be cleaned every day after use. At the same time lubricate thoroughly and tighten any loose screws.

Binding Setting: The boot must remain clamped to the ski during turns, but must detach before the force exerted on the leg becomes so great as to cause injury. Therefore, the binding setting is crucial. The setting must be tested every day before going on to the slopes as it can be affected by vibration, change of temperature or lack of proper maintenance.

In skiing more than any other sport proper conditioning before taking to the piste is quite essential to avoid injuries. Even so, most skiing injuries are to the lower limbs and include **strains and sprains** and the occasional **leg fracture.** Ankle and knee sprains are particularly common and are often caused by bad technique, inexperience in not being able to control the skis in an emergency, or bindings not detaching in time. Another common cause of leg injury is crossing skis, or actual collision with a tree, slalom gate or another skier. If immediately treated by a doctor, the healing time of these injuries can be dramatically reduced.

The thumb, fingers or shoulder are also susceptible to **dislocations**, particularly if a ski pole catches in a branch or other obstruction, or if the pole

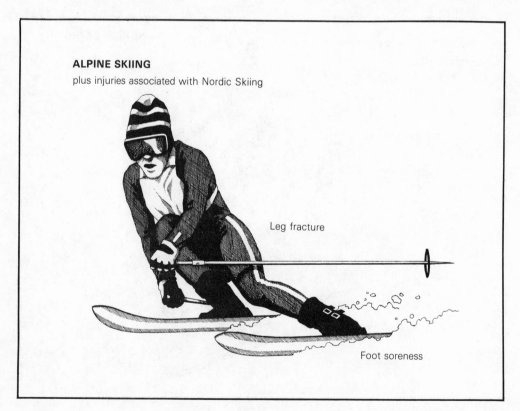

ALPINE SKIING
plus injuries associated with Nordic Skiing

Leg fracture

Foot soreness

straps catch on the hand. Hand injuries can also be caused by falling or collision. Sprained wrists in particular are common in the early stages of a skiing season, especially if there is little snow—beginners should wear mitts rather than gloves to save injury to fingers.

Muscle soreness, particularly of the arms, neck, shoulders and legs are characteristic of the early season. This soreness is aggravated by tension and the activity of swinging the ski poles. Taking a hot bath or shower and flexing the muscles under water should get rid of most of the soreness and subsequent stiffness. Massage, sauna and swimming in a heated pool are also highly beneficial alternatives.

Another common condition for the inexperienced or unfit skier is **lower back pain**, which is contributed to by weak abdominal muscles, tight hamstrings and stiff back muscles. Tension can heighten the condition. If the pain is acute see a doctor as the condition may be more severe than you had first thought. Otherwise treatment, as for muscle soreness, should do much to ease the discomfort. Carry out strength and flexibility exercises as soon as you are able. To help lessen the likelihood of lower back pain make sure that your preseason exercise routine includes ample exercises for strengthening the back and abdomen, and increasing the flexibility of the back and hamstrings.

Foot soreness is due to having ill-fitting boots. When buying ski boots, take the greatest care that they are comfortable and fit correctly. Remember that your entire week or weekend on the slopes could be ruined by badly fitting boots; it is therefore well worthwhile not relying on a borrowed or hired pair. Accustom the feet to the boots well ahead of use by wearing at home—but *do not* use them for going on long walks. Should you hire skis, make sure that the bindings fit your boots perfectly, and see also that they are correctly adjusted.

Artificial ski slopes have added a new injury to those normally associated with snow skiing. This is **burning and abrasions** resulting from a fall. Wear trousers, long sleeves and gloves, however hot the weather may be, to prevent the arms, hands and legs being skinned.

Sunburn and **snow blindness** can cause misery on the ski slopes. Ensure that you have barrier cream with you, and put it on before setting out. Sun goggles are an essential part of the equipment of any skier; some people take a spare pair in case of accidents.

Speed Skating

SPEED SKATING IS AN exhausting sport, requiring a very high standard of general fitness. Specifically, it calls for good heart and lung endurance; strength, especially in the body and legs; and flexibility in shoulders, arms and legs.

Alternative Sports: Every speed skater should attempt to maintain a high standard of general fitness throughout the off-season period. For this, running and jogging are hard to beat. The nearest comparable sport to speed skating, however, is cycling, which uses the same leg action; in fact, many cyclists take up speed skating as an alternative sport.

Warm-up: A thorough warm-up is essential. This usually takes the form of off-ice jogging followed by flexibility exercises, especially for the lower body and legs. Follow these with on-ice limbering exercises and skating movement practice.

SPEED SKATING FITNESS EXERCISES

Flexibility
F1. Side bends—hips and thighs
F2. Trunk Twists—trunk and neck
F4. Neck Rolls—neck
F7. Arm Circles—arms and upper trunk
F11. The Lunge—groin and thighs
F12. Hurdles—groin and thighs

Strength
S1. Push-Ups or Modified Push-Ups —body
S2. Pull-Ups—arms and shoulders
S9. "Bicycling"—abdomen
S10. Bent-Leg Sit-Ups—abdomen
S12. Squat Thrusts—thighs
S17. Bench Jumps—upper leg
S18. Shin Strengtheners—lower leg

In addition, weight training under supervision, especially for the body and legs.

Heart and Lung
Running   Cycling
Jogging   Ropework

In addition, a number of specific off-ice exercises have been devised for speed skaters:

Alternate Knee Dips: Stand erect, feet 12-15 inches apart, arms on hips. Lean to the left (avoid tilting either forward or backward), bending the left knee but keeping the right leg straight. Force the left knee as near the ground as you comfortably can, then straighten. Repeat on the other side. This is a good exercise for the knee and thigh.

Repetitions: 5 each side, increasing to 10

Sideways Skating (a variation of Alternate Knee Dips): On completion of the lean to the left, take the right leg across in front of the left leg, dipping down the body as you do so (in other words, simulate the speed skating leg movement). Return to the upright position, and repeat on the other side.

Thigh and Knee Circles: Stand erect, feet together, hands on hips. Bend both knees forward until you have adopted a half-squat position, then circle the knees around in a counterclockwise fashion. Keep the knees clasped together all the time. The body should remain erect.

Repetitions: 5 circles, increasing to 10

Bounce Jumps: Stand erect, feet together, hand on hips. Still with feet together, jump as high as you can. On landing, bend the knees and get as close to the ground as you can. The hands should touch the ground. Then spring up and repeat.

Repetitions: 5, increasing to 10

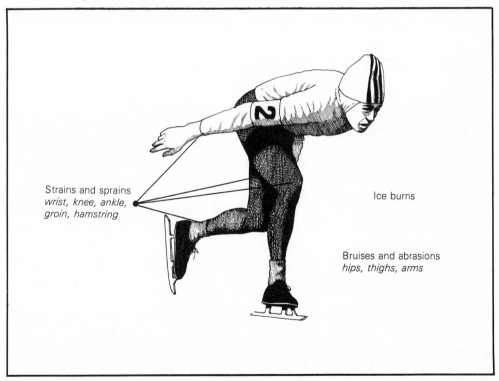

Strains and sprains
wrist, knee, ankle, groin, hamstring

Ice burns

Bruises and abrasions
hips, thighs, arms

HOME CIRCUIT
Preliminary warm-up
Jogging on the spot
Ropework, if appropriate
F2. Trunk Twists
S1. Push-Ups or Modified Push-Ups
Bounce Jumps
F11. The Lunge
S17. Bench Jumps
F7. Arm Circles
S12. Squat Thrusts
F1. Side Bends

SPEED SKATING INJURIES
The most common injuries in speed skating are **bruises and abrasions** caused by falling on the ice. The most vulnerable parts of the body for these are the hips, thighs and arms, and it is well worth while to wear long sleeves and gloves as a form of protection. **Ice burns**, caused by skidding along the ice, are also quite frequent.

Strains and sprains, particularly to the wrists, knees, ankles, groin and hamstrings are also quite common in the sport. These can be largely avoided by carrying out flexibility and strength exercises as part of the conditioning program and also completing a really thorough warm-up before taking part in a race or a training workout.

Figure Skating

FIGURE SKATING IS A SPORT requiring grace, precision and considerable athletic ability. Great stamina is not needed, but sustained effort and a high degree of concentration is called for during both short and long programs. This means that a high standard of general fitness is essential. Strength is needed, especially in the shoulders, arms, knees and ankles, and flexibility is required in the hips, shoulders, arms and legs.

Alternative Sports: Skating is unique in that it uses muscles that are not employed to any great extent in other sports; thus to overexercise at team or racquet sports could have an adverse effect on skating performance. The object of taking part in alternative sports, then, should be to maintain a reasonable standard of general fitness and basic conditioning. How strenuously to exercise off skates is an individual matter; each skater must learn to pace himself or herself accordingly. With this in mind, tennis, squash, jogging or running, and some light swimming are all useful alternative or off-season sports. Gymnastics, ballet and modern dance are also useful activities for cultivating the essential rhythm, flow and grace of figure skating. It must be said, however, that skating is still the best conditioner for skating.

Warm-Up: The obviously strenuous and sustained use of muscles that figure skating demands indicates that warming up is essential. However, coaches tend to have strong (and varying) views on the amount and form of warm-up necessary. Most skaters carry out simple limbering-up exercises before going on the ice. Once on the ice, more exercises (with emphasis on hips, shoulders, arms and legs) are carried out. These are usually followed by some forward and backward skating to loosen the muscles further and to help establish rhythm.

FIGURE SKATING FITNESS EXERCISES

F2. Trunk Twists—trunk and neck

F3. Alternate Toe Touches—back, shoulders and arms

F4. Neck Rolls—neck

F5. Shoulder Shrugs—shoulders

F7. Arm Circles—arms and upper body

F9. Wrist Shakes—wrists and hands

F13. Leg Swings—upper leg

Strength

S1. Push-Ups or Modified Push-Ups —body

S3. Two-Chair Push-Ups—arms and shoulders

S13. Sprinters—thighs

S16. Step-Ups—upper leg

S18. Shin Strengtheners—lower leg and ankle

S19. Calf Raises—lower leg and ankle

In addition, a useful skating exercise is **The Arch Strengthener:** Stand or sit with the feet on the ground. Pull up the arches of the feet and curl up the toes (either in or out of shoes), hold for 8–10 seconds, then relax. Repeat 3–5 times. This is an exercise that can be done almost anywhere at any time, and should be repeated 4–5 times a day.

Heart and Lung

Running

Jogging

Ropework

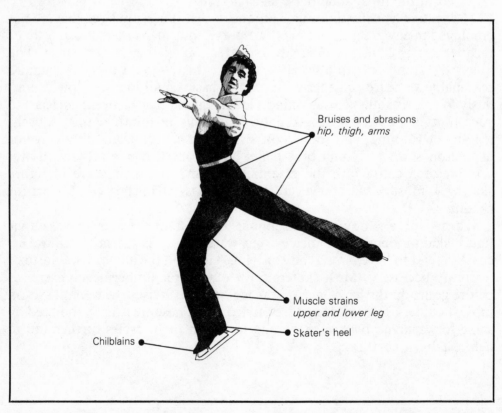

Bruises and abrasions
hip, thigh, arms

Muscle strains
upper and lower leg

Skater's heel

Chilblains

HOME CIRCUIT
Preliminary warm-up
Jogging on the spot
Ropework, if appropriate; otherwise
   jogging
F5. Shoulder Shrugs
F13. Leg Swings
S13. Sprinters
F2. Trunk Twists
S16. Step-Ups
F3. Alternate Toe Touches
S19. Calf Raises
F7. Arm Circles

FIGURE SKATING INJURIES
Bruises and abrasions are caused by falling on the ice and are treated as occupational hazards by most skaters. The hips, thighs and arms are particularly subject to these, as are the hands, and it is advisable to wear gloves whenever practicable.

Muscle strains, especially of the leg, are often due to inadequate warm-up. More severe ankle and foot problems are almost always due to having ill-designed or ill-fitting boots.

Skater's heel is an inflammation of the heel bursa brought about by wearing ill-fitting or too tightly-laced boots. Rest is the only satisfactory treatment here, although consequent swelling may be reduced by applying ice. Sponge padding under the heel will reduce the pain when walking.

Chilblains: Foot condition peculiar to ice skaters. These can be a painful nuisance as they cause the feet to swell which in turn makes the boots too tight. They are caused by coming off the ice and then immediately placing the feet near a radiator or fire.

Ice Hockey

ICE HOCKEY IS THE FASTEST, toughest and, to many, the most exciting team sport in the world. It is a contact sport played at a fierce pace and one requiring a very high degree of general fitness and all-around athletic ability. It calls for great stamina, explosive power and lightning fast reflexes and reactions. Skating skill is the first prerequisite.

Specifically, hockey requires a high level of heart and lung endurance; strength, especially in the body, arms, wrists and legs, and flexibility in the trunk, arms, wrists, legs and particularly the ankles.

Alternative Sports: Running, cycling, swimming and speed skating are all good stamina builders. Fast racquet sports such as squash and badminton, volleyball and handball are excellent for improving body coordination and reflexes.

Warm-Up: This should include jogging and stretching exercises off the ice, followed by on-the-ice practice including drills involving quick bursts of speed and puck passing.

ICE HOCKEY FITNESS EXERCISES

Flexibility

F1. Side Bends—hips and thighs
F2. Trunk Twists—trunk and neck
F3. Alternate Toe Touches—back, shoulders and arms
F6. Wing Stretchers—shoulders
F7. Arm Circles—arms and upper body
F9. Wrist Shakes—wrists
F11. The Lunge—groin and thigh
F14. Knee Pulls—lower leg

Strength

S1. Push-Ups or Modified Push-Ups —body
S2. Pull-Ups—arms and shoulders
S5. Broomstick Rolls—wrists and hands
S10. Bent-Leg Sit-Ups—abdomen
S12. Squat Thrusts—thighs
S16. Step-Ups—upper leg
S17. Bench Jumps—upper leg
S19. Calf Raises—lower leg

In addition, weight training under supervision, especially for the body, arms, wrists and legs.

Speed-skating exercises (*see* p. 186) are excellent for stretching and strengthening the skating muscles.

Heart and Lung
Running, especially Fartlek and interval training
Swimming
Ropework
Cycling
Speed skating

HOME CIRCUIT
Preliminary warm-up
Running on the spot
Ropework, if appropriate; otherwise jogging

S1. Push-Ups or Modified Push-Ups
F2. Trunk Twists
F11. The Lunge
S10. Bent-Leg Sit-Ups
F3. Alternate Toe Touches
S2. Pull-Ups
F1. Side Bends
S12. Squat Thrusts

ICE HOCKEY INJURIES
As would be expected in a very fast contact game such as ice hockey, injuries are inclined to be extensive and can be severe.

Bruising, either from the stick, puck, or collision with the side boards or another player is a very common ice hockey injury. Most vulnerable are the upper legs and the arms. Hands,

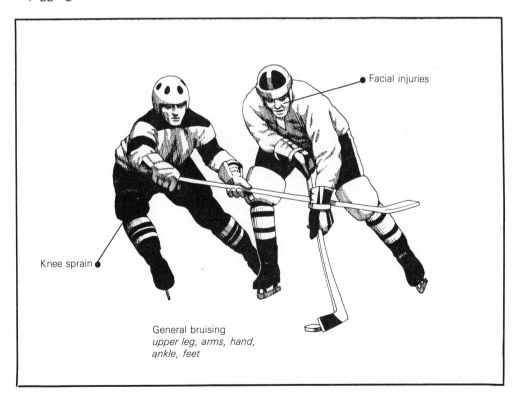

Facial injuries

Knee sprain

General bruising
upper leg, arms, hand, ankle, feet

despite the protection afforded by gloves, are also subject to considerable bruising, as are the ankles and feet—although skating boots do give a measure of protection.

Cuts and abrasions, as well as **ice burns,** are frequent ice hockey injuries and these can be severe.

Knee sprain is a frequent affliction of the amateur ice hockey player and is usually due to a sudden twist, turn or fall. Exercises for strengthening the upper leg muscles during the conditioning program, as well as thorough warming-up before a game, should do much to lessen the likelihood of knee strain.

Facial injuries: In amateur ice hockey the helmet wards off many head injuries. However, a direct blow to the face from either a puck or stick can cause cut lips and lost teeth (unless a mouth guard is worn). In extreme cases a broken jaw could result. In the professional game headgear is frequently not worn, and as a result head and facial injuries ranging from bleeding or broken noses to concussion are rife.

Roller Skating

ROLLER SKATING IS A SPORT that requires considerable strength and flexibility, but above all it calls for lightning-fast reactions and reflexes. Pair, dance and figure roller skaters do not require great powers of heart and lung endurance, but sustained short-term effort is needed for periods of up to 5 minutes at a time. Speed roller skating, on the other hand, demands considerable stamina, while hockey skaters must have good body strength as well in order to play their part in a most vigorous contact sport.

Specific fitness for roller skaters involves strong legs and trunk, and flexibility in hips, shoulders, knees and ankles. Pair skaters need additional strength in the diaphragm, shoulders and arms.

Alternative Sports: As ice skating, roller skating uses muscles that are not employed to any great extent in other sports. Thus to overexercise them at team and racquet games could have an adverse effect. How strenuously to exercise off skates is an individual matter; roller skaters must learn to pace themselves. The need is to maintain a high general standard of fitness. For this, jogging and running and light swimming are useful alternative pursuits.

In addition to the physical requirements of the sport, roller skaters have to have a clear head in order to be able to cope with situations that arise in a sport which is one of the fastest on earth.

Warm-Up: To roller skate with "cold" muscles is asking for strains and sprains. Before putting on their skates, roller skaters usually perform gentle flexibility exercises, with the emphasis on hips, shoulders, knees and ankles.

ROLLER SKATING FITNESS
EXERCISES

When done with care and in moderation, the following exercises will be found to be of use for those with particular weaknesses. For speed roller skaters, especially distance skaters, stamina and leg strength are essential.

Flexibility
F2. Trunk Twists—trunk and neck
F3. Alternate Toe Touches—back, shoulders and arms
F4. Neck Rolls—neck
F5. Shoulder Shrugs—shoulders
F9. Wrist Shakes—wrist and hands
F13. Leg Swings—upper legs

Strength
S1. Push-Ups or Modified Push-Ups —body
S3. Two-Chair Push-Ups—arms and shoulders
S16. Step-Ups—upper legs (also a very good heart and lung exercise for roller skaters)
S19. Calf Raises—lower leg

Speed skaters should add:
S11. Half Squats—thighs

S12. Squat Thrusts
S15. Leg Raises—upper leg

Heart and Lung
Running
Jogging
Ropework

HOME CIRCUIT
Preliminary warm-up
Jogging on the spot
Ropework, if appropriate; otherwise jogging
F5. Shoulder Shrugs
S3. Two-Chair Push-Ups
F3. Alternate Toe Touches
S16. Step-Ups
F4. Neck Rolls

Speed skaters should add:
S11. Half Squats
S12. Squat Thrusts

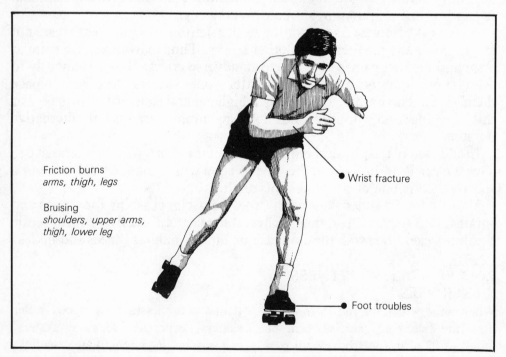

Friction burns
arms, thigh, legs

Bruising
shoulders, upper arms, thigh, lower leg

Wrist fracture

Foot troubles

ROLLER SKATING INJURIES

The most common roller skating injuries are **bruises**, particularly to the shoulder, upper arm, thigh and lower leg, and **friction burns**, to which the arm, thigh and leg are very susceptible.

Fractures are caused when a skater falls. Wrist fractures, the most frequent fracture, can occur when a skater falls on a bent wrist or puts out a hand to save a fall. Injuries resulting from falls are often made much worse because the skater is tense and has not been taught how to fall (for this aspect of roller skating some martial arts, such as judo and aikido, are invaluable.)

As with ice skating **foot trouble** is quite frequent in roller skating. The bottoms of the feet in particular—the heel ball and the sole—are most vulnerable. Foot hygiene is essential and many skaters use foot deodorants and refreshers, which contain a hardening agent. Care must also be taken not to lace the boots too tightly.

A good general tip for foot care is to bathe the feet in salty water after skating, which is very soothing. It is also advisable not to put on talcum or other foot powder before roller skating, as this tends to allow the feet to slip in the boot, which may cause blisters.

Skateboarding

SKATEBOARDING TAKES TWO basic forms. By far the most popular and widespread version of the sport is recreational skateboarding, done by a large number of youngsters. At a different level is competitive skateboarding, which is fast becoming a recognized sport; this requires stamina, strength and agility of a very high order so as to achieve the essential rhythmic flow which is the hallmark of high-class skateboarding.

Recreational skateboarding requires little conditioning; the natural strengths and agility of the youngster are usually sufficient. Competitive skateboarding, on the other hand, calls for a high standard of general fitness, including considerable heart and lung endurance; strength, especially in the back and upper and lower legs; and flexibility in the lower parts of the body, as well as in arms and legs.

Alternative Sports: Running and swimming aid general stamina improvement. Nordic skiing, alpine skiing and ice skating assist with the essential balance and timing required for the sport, as do martial arts such as karate, judo and aikido. Basketball, squash and gymnastics improve general suppleness.

Warm-Up: Jogging and gentle flexibility exercises are useful in toning the muscles and lowering tension, which is a primary cause of injury.

SKATEBOARDING FITNESS EXERCISES

Flexibility
F1. Side Bends—hips and thighs
F2. Trunk Twists—trunk and neck
F7. Arm Circles—arms, upper trunk
F11. The Lunge—groin and thighs
F13. Leg Swings—upper legs
F14. Knee Pulls—lower legs

Strength
S1. Push-Ups or Modified Push-Ups —body
S9. "Bicycling"—abdomen
S10. Bent-Leg Sit-Ups—abdomen
S13. Sprinters—thighs
S17. Bench Jumps—upper leg
S18. Shin Strengtheners—lower leg

198

Heart and Lung
Running   Jogging   Ropework

HOME CIRCUIT
Preliminary warm-up
Jogging on the spot
Ropework, if appropriate
S1. Push-Ups or Modified Push-Ups
F2. Trunk Twists
S9. "Bicycling"
F7. Arm Circles
S17. Bench Jumps
F14. Knee Pulls

SKATEBOARDING INJURIES
After bicycling, skateboarding is the most prevalent sport in which children are injured. Adults are certainly not immune, and accidents arise when a parent or helpful friend thinks he can skateboard, and finds, painfully, that he cannot.

Bruises, cuts and abrasions, particularly to the arms and legs, are quite common. **Sprained wrists and ankles** are also not infrequent. **Fractures** may be sustained, usually to the wrist, forearm, elbow, thumb, fingers, or the collarbone. When these occur, medical attention is essential.

Protection: Serious injury is largely prevented by wearing protective equipment, particularly a light-weight helmet and elbow and knee pads. It is also advisable to wear gloves, long trousers and rubber-soled shoes. Take steps to ensure that protective gear is kept in good condition, and make sure that the nonslip tape on top of the skateboard remains intact.

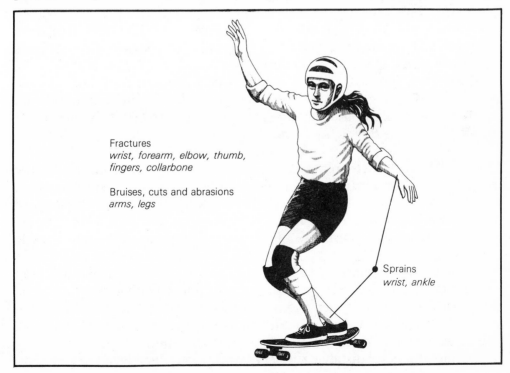

Fractures
wrist, forearm, elbow, thumb, fingers, collarbone

Bruises, cuts and abrasions
arms, legs

Sprains
wrist, ankle

Running
Sprinting and Distance

SPRINTING (100, 200, 400 meters) depends on a combination of leg speed and length of stride. This calls for very strong legs to give the necessary impetus in the powerful extended leg drive, but it also calls for strong arms and shoulders to provide body balance. It is essentially an explosive event demanding quick reflexes and perfect coordination of movement. The real secret of successful sprinting lies in the ability to run with reduced tension—a blend of mental approach, personal confidence and physical suppleness.

Specific fitness for the sprinter involves a high level of heart and lung endurance; strength in the thighs and hips, knees and ankles, as well as in the shoulders and upper arms; flexibility, especially in the legs, body, shoulders and neck, which is the source of a lot of tension in the runner.

Alternative Sports: Running, jogging and ropework are useful stamina builders. Mobility sports such as basketball, volleyball and badminton are excellent, particularly as a change from running training. Gymnastics is invaluable for improving all-round suppleness.

DISTANCE RUNNING combines power with heart and lung endurance. The longer-distance and marathon runners (over 1,500 meters) require stamina above all else; middle-distance runners (800 and 1,500 meters) neglect speed at their peril. However, all need to acquire an economical technique, one that makes maximum use of the body's oxygen intake and muscle endurance.

As a general rule, the easy stride of the distance runner calls for less pure leg strength than is needed by the sprinter; the relaxed swinging action of the arms demands less shoulder and arm strength. Nevertheless, a very high general fitness level is required of the distance runner, as well as considerable mental discipline for what is an intensely lonely sport.

Specific fitness for distance runners involves very high levels of heart and lung endurance; strength in the abdomen, back, shoulders and legs (weak calves and ankles tend toward a flat-footed run); and flexibility in the body and back, hips and legs.

Alternative Sports: The necessary capacity for sustained running over long distances is built up by extensive training runs—up to 10 miles and more, and much of it cross-country. This leaves little time for alternative forms of exercise; however cycling and walking as well as ropework are possible alternatives. Also useful, as a mental change as much as for their inherent value in promoting mobility and general suppleness, are squash, badminton, basketball and volleyball.

RUNNING INJURIES

Many running injuries can be avoided with proper conditioning and thorough warm-up before a training session or competition, *and* thorough warm-down afterwards. Nevertheless, running injuries are quite frequent and almost always, except in the case of a fall or accident, involve the lower limbs. These include **plantar fasciitis** and **heel spurs** of the foot, both helped considerably by wearing well-padded shoes with a good heel lift. **Blisters,** especially for distance runners, is another

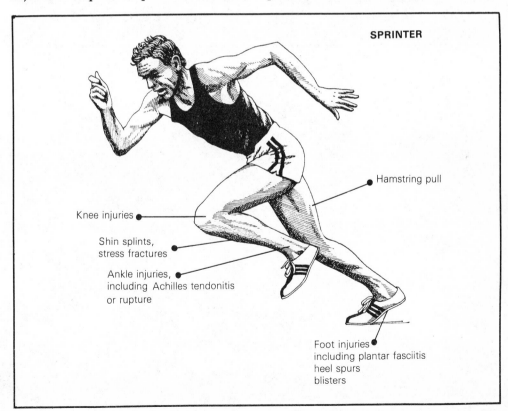

SPRINTER

Hamstring pull

Knee injuries

Shin splints, stress fractures

Ankle injuries, including Achilles tendonitis or rupture

Foot injuries including plantar fasciitis heel spurs blisters common foot complaint, and foot hardening with alcohol or a skin-hardening agent is essential at the start of the season or after a long lay-off.

Ankle injuries embrace soreness and sprains—strengthening and flexibility exercises combined with proper warm-up should materially assist in preventing these. The **Achilles tendon** is also very susceptible to injury, either from **tendonitis** or **rupture,** either partial or complete.

The shin suffers from **shin splints** or **stress fractures,** often brought on by running on very hard ground, particularly at the start of the season.

The **knee** is also subject to injury, often through running on hard ground at the start of the season or because of poor running technique. Structurally weak feet can be responsible as well. Strengthening and flexibility exercises will help here; if chronic trouble develops seek advice from a foot specialist.

Hamstring pull can be totally incapacitating. Imbalance between the relative muscle strengths of the quadriceps at the front of the thigh and the hamstrings at the back is often responsible. This can be remedied by balanced strength and flexibility exercises.

Runners are also subject to **general muscle soreness, cramps** and **the stitch. Runner's nipple,** a condition which causes sore nipples due to the constant rubbing of clothing during a run, can also cause discomfort. Protective tape is the best answer here.

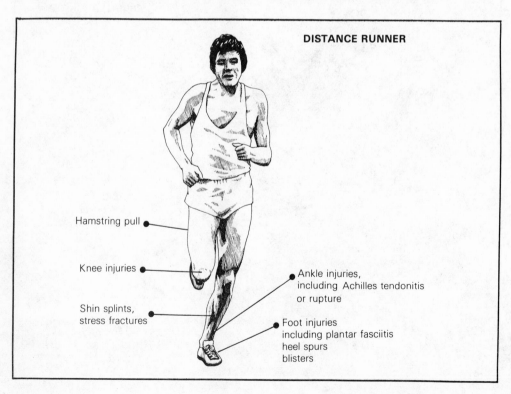

DISTANCE RUNNER

Hamstring pull

Knee injuries

Shin splints, stress fractures

Ankle injuries, including Achilles tendonitis or rupture

Foot injuries including plantar fasciitis heel spurs blisters

Hurdling

HURDLING REQUIRES the speed of the sprinter, as well as suppleness, strength, stamina and fine overall body coordination. In addition, the hurdler must be a good judge of distance, possess a sense of balance and more than a little courage.

Hurdling should conform as near as possible to the normal action of running, and there should be a minimum break in rhythm and cadence. This calls for strong legs to provide the powerful drive at the start of the take-off stride and a high degree of hip mobility as the take-off leg folds over in crossing the hurdle.

Specific fitness for hurdling involves a high level of heart and lung endurance; strength, particularly in the legs, hips, abdomen, arms and shoulders; flexibility in the legs and hips as well as in the back, groin, hamstrings and arms.

Alternative Sports: Running, jogging, swimming and ropework are all good for stamina building. Team games such as basketball and soccer are sometimes popular, but a number of coaches prefer their athletes not to run the risk of injury in such sports. Tennis, volleyball, squash, badminton and racquetball are all useful agility sports. Gymnastics is excellent for all-round suppleness.

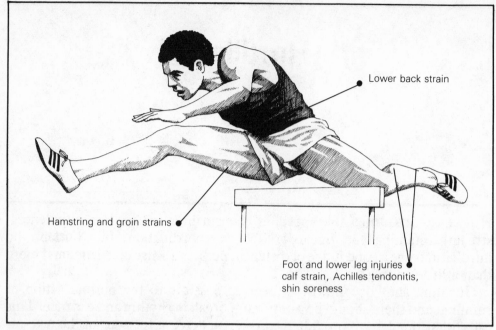

Lower back strain

Hamstring and groin strains

Foot and lower leg injuries
calf strain, Achilles tendonitis,
shin soreness

HURDLING INJURIES

Many hurdling injuries can be avoided with proper conditioning and thorough warm-up before training or competition. Nevertheless, hurdling is quite an injury-prone sport.

Hamstring and groin strains are quite frequent and require total rest before the athlete is fit enough to hurdle again.

Foot and lower leg injuries, such as **calf strain** and **Achilles tendonitis** are quite common. In addition, **shin soreness** is becoming more frequent with hurdlers on some of the newer types of track due to the recoil or spring-back of the surface after the runner's weight has come down on it.

The **lower back** is also vulnerable to strain during hurdling, but this is usually due to failing to warm-up properly, especially in cold weather.

Race Walking

RACE WALKING ESSENTIALLY requires a great deal of stamina for either the 20 km "sprint" or endurance races of 50 km or longer. Although it eats up the ground, the rolling technique of race walking is extremely wearying, especially for those who are not at the very peak of fitness; thus a high degree of all-round conditioning is also obligatory.

The essence of race walking is that the stride should be smooth and rhythmical, with an easy natural arm action. The supporting leg must be fully straightened to give a strong forward drive, and the posture must be erect—if tilted backward, the spine may be jarred and the stride length shortened; if forward, the stride length will also be shortened and the walker will have trouble straightening the leading leg.

Specific fitness for the race walker involves a very high degree of heart and lung endurance; strength in the legs (especially the thighs and ankles), the abdomen and back; and flexibility in the hips and legs (especially the hamstrings) as well as in the shoulders, upper back and neck. The latter three are principal sources of tension in the walker, and this can lead to reduced performance and unnecessary vulnerability to injury.

Alternative Sports: Walking is, of course, the principal heart and lung exercise for the walker. As a variation some walkers choose to do cross-country running, especially if there is ice on the roads. Others prefer swimming. Certain games such as squash, badminton and volleyball are good for general mobility. Gymnastics is invaluable for promoting overall suppleness.

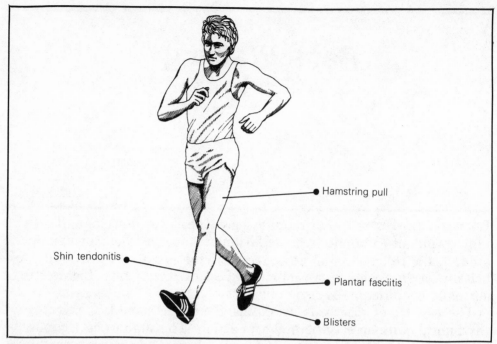

Hamstring pull

Shin tendonitis

Plantar fasciitis

Blisters

RACE WALKING INJURIES

The **hamstrings** are a frequent site of injury in race walking. The walking technique calls for particularly strong quadriceps muscles at the front of the upper leg and this strength is often at the expense of the hamstrings at the back of the thigh; as a result of this imbalance hamstring pulls are quite common. Balanced flexibility and strength exercises for the two muscle groups should do much to reduce the incidence of hamstring injuries.

The foot is also subject to injury in race walking. **Plantar fasciitis** on the sole of the foot can be a grave handicap and is aggravated or caused by walking on very hard surfaces before the runner is fully conditioned. Well-padded shoes should do much to help here.

Tendonitis of the front of the shin is another common walking injury and is due to increasing distance and speed before the walker is really ready or because of inadequate warm-up.

Long and Triple Jump

LONG JUMPING essentially requires speed, spring and strength. The long jump movement must flow—from the approach run with its emphasis on speed rather than stride length, to the explosive take-off from the board, the balanced flight and controlled landing. The speed that is called for is the speed of the sprinter—indeed many long jumpers are first-class sprinters—with a consistent stride length and smooth acceleration. This calls for strong legs—especially the knees and ankles—and a strong trunk and abdomen to give stability to the erect jumping position. It also calls for power in the hip, knee and ankle to give maximum drive from the board. And without an essential degree of timing and aggression the long-jumper will get nowhere.

Triple jumping calls for the approach speed to be conserved for all three phases of the jump. This requires a perfect use of controlled speed, ideal body balance and body coordination so as to create what is, in effect, one continuous rhythmic movement. Strong legs are needed for the initial lift-off from the board and the subsequent contacts with the ground.

Specific fitness for long and triple jumpers involves a high level of heart and lung endurance; strength, particularly in the legs (especially knees and ankles), the trunk, abdomen and hips; and flexibility in the back, hips, knees and ankles.

Alternative Sports: Running, jogging, swimming and ropework are all good stamina builders. Of track and field athletic events, hurdling and sprinting are particularly beneficial. Games such as squash, tennis and basketball are excellent for all-round agility. Gymnastics are an invaluable aid to general suppleness.

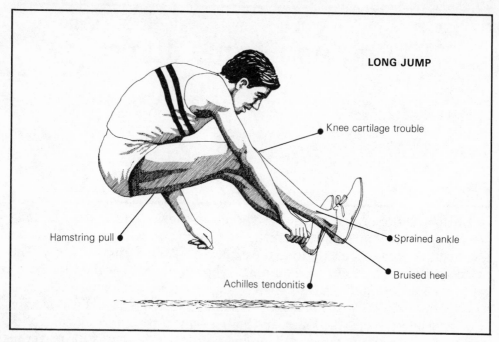

LONG JUMP

Knee cartilage trouble

Hamstring pull

Sprained ankle

Bruised heel

Achilles tendonitis

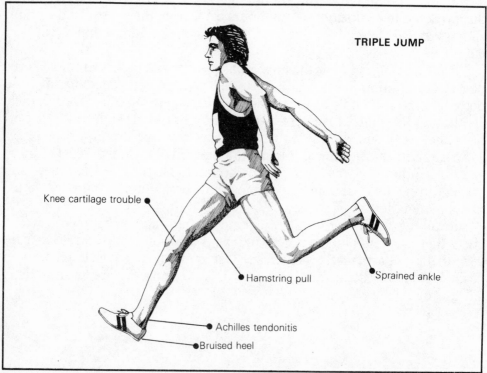

TRIPLE JUMP

Knee cartilage trouble

Hamstring pull

Sprained ankle

Achilles tendonitis

Bruised heel

LONG AND TRIPLE JUMPING INJURIES

The long and triple jumper is suscept-ible to both the injuries of the sprinter and those more specifically associated with the movements of his own sport. Injuries are mainly to the leg and these include **bruised heels**, **Achilles ten-donitis** and **twisted ankles**. The latter often occur on take-off or are due to running on a rough or ill-prepared approach.

Cartilage trouble with the knee is another long and triple jumping injury. **Hamstring pulls** are also quite frequent and are often due to overexercising in cold weather without a good warm-up.

Most of these injuries can be avoided with a full program of conditioning which includes flexing and strengthen-ing exercises for the vulnerable areas, a really thorough warm-up before prac-tice or competition, and a good warm-down afterward.

High Jump

HIGH JUMPING is essentially the coordination of speed and spring. It calls for a very high standard of general fitness and considerable stamina. Although the lower body must be considered the power house in the high jump, with strong and flexible legs required for the explosive upwards lift at take-off, the arm swing is necessary to add momentum to the leap, and the whole demands excellent overall body coordination.

There are two principal versions of the high jump today: the straddle and the Fosbury flop, which first came to notice in the late 1960s at the hands of Dick Fosbury and has revolutionized high jumping, particularly women's high jumping. The principal physical differences between the two styles is that the straddle requires the greater strength and a very disciplined rhythm in the approach; and the Fosbury demands more speed in what is usually a curved approach run.

Specific fitness for high jumping involves a high level of heart and lung endurance; strength in the whole body, particularly in the lower back and hips, as well as in the shoulders and the jumping muscles of the leg (the quadriceps and hamstrings). Flexibility is called for in the hips, back, shoulders and legs.

Alternative Sports: Running, jogging, swimming and ropework are excellent for stamina building. Other track and field events such as hurdling, short sprints, the pole vault, and long and triple jump are also useful for the high jumper. Volleyball, basketball and squash are good alternative or off-season sports, although many coaches frown on athletes playing contact games which might lead to serious injury. Gymnastics and trampoline work aid general suppleness.

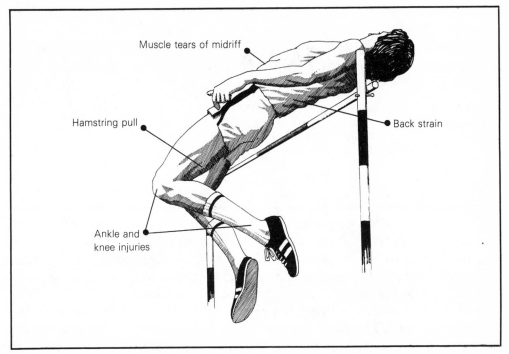

Muscle tears of midriff

Hamstring pull

Back strain

Ankle and
knee injuries

HIGH JUMPING INJURIES

The **hamstrings** are very vulnerable to strains in both styles of high jumping, as are the **ankles and knees** in the run-up. To help prevent hamstring trouble, it is important to maintain a balance in strength between the quadriceps muscles at the front of the thigh, and the hamstrings at the back.

Straddle jumpers are prone to jarring of the foot, which can lead to **heel trouble** and also **soreness** at the base of the toes.

Fosbury jumpers are particularly vulnerable to **muscle tears in the midriff** and **back strain**.

The scissors jump, which is often used to train high jumpers, can lead to **strain in the stomach muscles**.

It is quite essential that the high jumper carry out extensive flexibility and strengthening exercises for all those parts of the body subject to strain. It is important also to carry out a proper warm-down routine after a training session or competition, to avoid muscle soreness and reduce the risk of subsequent injury.

Hammer

HAMMER THROWING REQUIRES stamina, mobility, agility, good body co-ordination, balance and footwork as well as a great deal of skill. It also requires strength—in the legs and lower body in order to able to turn fast, but also all-round strength to maintain the rhythm and flow of the rotations and then the final release, in one continuous movement.

The sequence of the throw indicates the specific physical needs of the hammer thrower. The arms and wrists come into play at first to set in motion the wind-ups or swings; thereafter, until final release, they act as little more than extensions of the hammer. Hammer-throwing power emanates from the lower trunk and legs, but the key to successful hammer throwing lies in the hips, which must be strong and flexible. Until the final whip-lash release, the upper trunk merely serves to help increase the centrifugal effect of the body turns on the hammer.

Specific fitness for hammer throwing involves a good standard of heart and lung endurance allied with strength, particularly in the lower body, legs and above all in the hips; and flexibility in the abdominal region, lower back and lower legs, as well as an overall suppleness.

Alternative Sports: Running, jogging, swimming, rope climbing and weight training are very good stamina builders, as is ropework generally. Certain track and field athletic events are also good for the hammer thrower, such as hurdling, the pole vault and jumping—high, long and triple. Very active games such as squash, basketball and volleyball all help increase speed and suppleness.

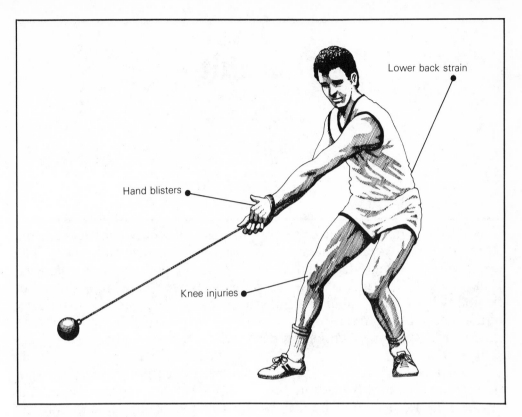

Lower back strain

Hand blisters

Knee injuries

HAMMER-THROWING INJURIES

Hammer-throwing injuries are largely related to two main aspects of the sport: the turning of a heavy body in a small circle, and the actual effort of the throw itself.

Knee injuries—varying from **tendonitis** to severe sprain and even cartilage trouble can occur as a result of the very tight turns the hammer thrower must perform. Flexibility and strengthening exercises during conditioning, as well as a thorough warm-up and warm-down before and after practice or competition, render these injuries less likely.

Lower back strain is caused by the whole throwing movement, but particularly by the release. The injury can be persistent and a severe handicap. On first feeling lower back strain it is essential to see a doctor straight away.

Hand blisters are an occupational injury to the hammer thrower. It will help to wear thicker gloves for training and thin ones during actual competition. But this is only a partial preventative and most throwers learn to live through blister pain.

Shot Put

SHOT PUTTING (also known as weight putting) is not only a matter of brute strength exerted by men and women of mountainous size and power. The event calls for a high degree of specific strength, particularly in the legs, back, shoulders, arms, hands and fingers, as well as a high degree of flexibility in the hips, shoulders and arms in particular. The essential power of the shot putter comes through the application of strength combined with speed, and this only works properly when there is perfect body co-ordination.

The sequence of the throw indicates the specific physical needs of the shot putter. First is a massive leg and hip drive, followed by the glide across the circle. This is succeeded by a powerful rotation of hips and shoulders, ending with the faster drive through the shoulders, the arms, wrists and finally the fingers. All-important is the flow of the throw and its rhythmical progression, which is literally a ripple of muscle power.

Specific fitness for the shot putter, therefore, involves a fair degree of heart and lung endurance and a high standard of general fitness. Strength is essential, the over-all body "brute" strength of the very big athlete and the specific strengths of his sport. Flexibility in the hips, shoulders, arms, wrists and fingers to provide the suppleness necessary in the essential flow of the putting action, and for rotation of the body before the explosive release.

Alternative Sports: Running, jogging and ropework are all popular stamina builders. Team games such as rugby, soccer handball and basketball help the athlete to acquire speed and strength; racquet sports such as squash are generally too jarring for a heavy body. Judo is excellent for general body suppleness.

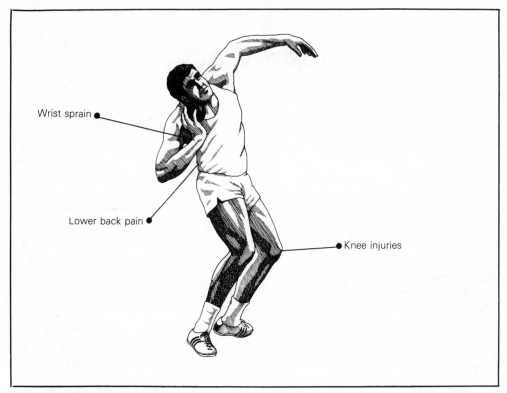

Wrist sprain

Lower back pain

Knee injuries

SHOT PUTTING INJURIES

Lower back pain is a condition shot or weight putters are inclined to suffer from due to the intense twisting motion of the lower body which they must use in the throw. Intensive flexibility and strengthening exercises are essential in helping to prevent this.

Wrist strain is another quite frequent injury and usually occurs on the final phase of the throw. Once again, intensive wrist flexibility and strengthening exercises are an intregral part of the conditioning program for the shot putter.

Knee injuries, including cartilage trouble, sometimes occur during weight-training sessions, which are an intregal part of a shot putter's fitness program.

Pole Vault

POLE VAULTING REQUIRES, above all else, supreme all-around fitness and strength. It is a very exhausting event needing speed, spring, body coordination and timing. It also calls for courage of a very high order, and very considerable aggression.

The take-off is a springing movement executed with great power and involving a powerful leg action designed to gain sufficient momentum for the rest of the vaulting movement. The "rock-back" that follows—when the vaulter tucks in the legs close to the pole—calls for powerful use of the abdominal muscles. When the catapulting motion of the pole begins to straighten it out, the vaulter must then perform what is virtually a handstand at the end of the pole. This calls for powerful arm and shoulder action to pull up the body. The spiral, twisting action that follows forces the feet and then the vaulter's whole body over the bar (which is considerably higher than the hands on the pole) and calls for great strength and immense flexibility in the back, shoulders and arms.

Specific fitness for pole vaulting, therefore, involves a high level of general fitness and heart and lung endurance, great strength, especially in the abdominal muscles and those of the back, shoulders and arms; and flexibility in the body—particularly the back and hips, shoulders, arms and knees.

Alternative Sports: Running, jogging, swimming and ropework are all good for stamina building. Weight lifting is good for general strength building, gymnastics is excellent for promoting all-round body suppleness. Certain track and field events are also useful for the pole vaulter, in particular sprints and the long and triple-jump. Other beneficial games are squash, badminton, basketball and volleyball.

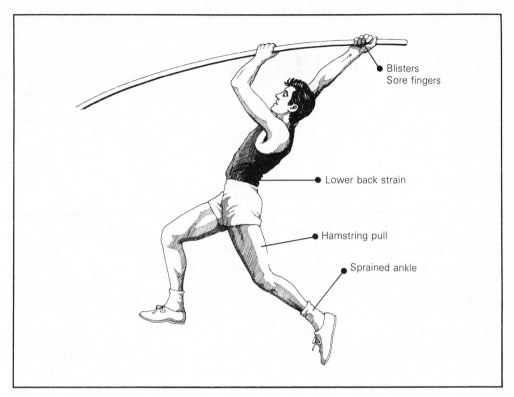

Blisters
Sore fingers

Lower back strain

Hamstring pull

Sprained ankle

POLE VAULTING INJURIES

The most severe injuries are caused when the pole breaks. Modern poles are extremely delicate and very prone to break in the course of a jump if they are previously damaged; when they do, the vaulter is likely to suffer arm or back injuries.

Hamstrings are particularly vulnerable to pulls during the run-up. Imbalance between the relative muscle strengths of the quadriceps muscles at the front of the thigh and the hamstrings at the back are often the cause. It is important to ensure that balanced strengthening and flexibility exercises are carried out.

for these muscle groups are carried out.

Sprained ankles are also fairly frequent in the pole vault. This can take place if the run-up is rough or ill-prepared, but a more usual cause is if the vaulter treads in the box after a stall out.

The **lower back** is also quite likely to suffer strain during the vault, especially if the vaulter finds himself too close to the bar during the vault or at take-off. Flexibility and strengthening exercises in the conditioning program should do much to help prevent lower back strain. A very useful exercise is hanging from a pull-up bar.

Discus

DISCUS THROWING REQUIRES the athlete to be fast, mobile and very strong; the throwing action is essentially a balance between strength and speed.

As with many field events, throwing the discus involves a ripple of muscle power, a rhythmic flowing motion from the leg through the muscles of the trunk, the shoulders, the arms and lastly the wrists, hands and fingers in the final sling-like release of the discus. The key to successful discus throwing lies in the leg and hip drive when the shoulders and hips must rotate together. The whole movement of throwing the discus requires strength, both general and specific, speed, skill and mobility. A special physical feature of discus throwing however is the powerful start and the almost immediate stop within the confines of a very small circle; this places considerable strain on the lower legs.

Specific fitness for discus throwing, therefore, involves a reasonable level of heart and lung endurance; strength, especially in the back, abdomen, ankles and knee joints, hips, shoulders and arms; and flexibility in the hips, shoulders, arms, wrists and legs—particularly in the ankle and knee.

Alternative Sports: Running, jogging, swimming and ropework are all good for stamina building. Squash, tennis and table tennis are useful alternative sports to speed up reflexes and as a general aid to suppleness. Basketball and volleyball are excellent in promoting speed combined with balance. Most discus throwers are also versatile athletes, especially in other field events.

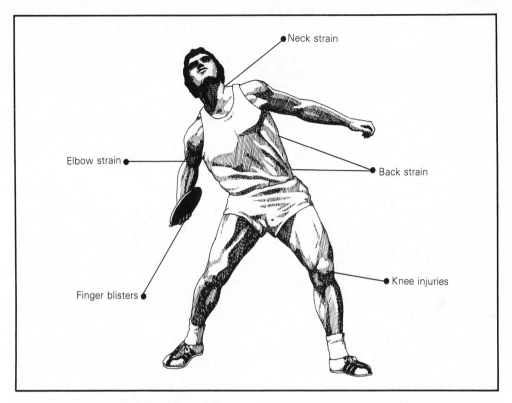

Neck strain

Elbow strain

Back strain

Knee injuries

Finger blisters

DISCUS THROWING INJURIES

The rotational movement involved in throwing the discus places considerable strain on many parts of the body.

The **knee** is particularly vulnerable, and knee injuries from **mild twists** to **severe cartilage** trouble do occur. The **back**, particularly the middle and upper back and the **neck** are also prone to injury during the rotational movement. This can lead to **disc trouble**, but even the mildest strain in this part of the body unless dealt with promptly and professionally can persist and recur and be a continuing handicap to the discus thrower. Intensive flexibility and strengthening exercises for all parts of the back and legs are essential if these injuries are to be avoided.

Strain of the elbow in the final release of the discus also occurs and can be very troublesome. Flexibility and strengthening exercises for the elbow and wrists are important in the discus thrower's fitness program.

Finger blisters are another common discus throwing complaint.

Javelin

JAVELIN THROWING REQUIRES a blend of speed in the initial approach run, power (especially in the legs) and a final flinging motion of the arm. To combine these ingredients demands first of all a high standard of general fitness together with considerable stamina and power, stride length, speed, specific strength, as well as suppleness, all molded together through perfect body coordination.

The run-up length varies between 80 to 120 feet, but at the end the javelin thrower must be accelerating. The speed generated in the run is increased by the final flinging motion of the javelin, but this itself is generated by rotational power from the hips allied with a rolling action by the shoulder and culminating in a whiplash effort of the arm. The whole must constitute a continuous, flowing movement.

Specific fitness for the javelin thrower, therefore, involves good heart and lung endurance; strength in the body, shoulders, arms, wrists, fingers and legs; and flexibility in hips, shoulders, arms, elbows, wrists, fingers and legs.

Alternative Sports: Running, jogging, swimming and ropework are all good for stamina building. Certain track and field athletic events are also useful for the javelin thrower, in particular hurdling, sprinting, and the long and triple jump. Basketball, handball, volleyball and squash are all excellent for promoting fitness and speed.

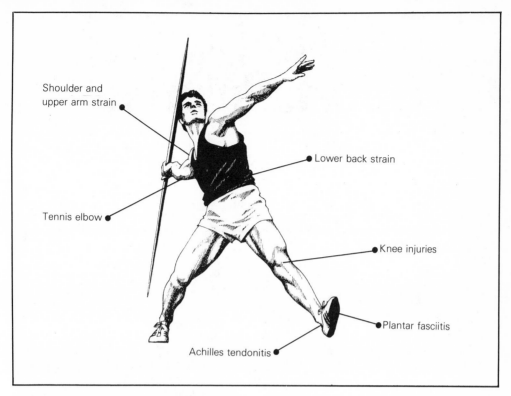

Shoulder and upper arm strain

Lower back strain

Tennis elbow

Knee injuries

Plantar fasciitis

Achilles tendonitis

JAVELIN THROWING INJURIES

Tennis Elbow is a common complaint with javelin throwers. It is particularly prevalent at the start of the season, and can also be caused by bad technique. For treatment and ways to ease the pain, *see* Tennis, pp. 132–133.

The **foot and lower leg** are also vulnerable during the run-up and particularly in the final flinging action of the javelin throw. Injuries to these parts of the body include **plantar fasciitis** in the sole of the foot, **Achilles tendonitis** and **knee ailments** varying from **mild strain** to severe **cartilage trouble.** Many lower leg injuries can be largely prevented by carrying out thorough flexibility and strengthening exercises during the conditioning program. **Plantar fasciitis** can often be prevented by building up the heel in the running shoe, or using arch supports.

The rotational movement involved in the javelin throw places considerable strain on the body, particularly the lower back, and **lower back strain** is a common javelin-throwing complaint. Flexibility and strengthening exercises are invaluable in helping to prevent this injury, as they are to **shoulder** and **upper arm strain** caused in the final fling of the javelin.

PART III
Sports Injuries

No WRITTEN WORDS are a substitute for on-the-spot medical advice, just as no book can give complete guidance on the symptoms or treatment of injuries. Every injured person is a law unto himself or herself, and every injury is unique—however minor.

In spite of this, there are many common athletic injuries, ailments and conditions that can be dealt with by home treatment. The first two sections of Part III discuss a wide range of such injuries—their symptoms, treatment and prevention. A final section is devoted to first aid advice for emergencies that may arise on the sports field.

If there is one aspect above all others that has come out of my discussions with coaches, trainers and athletes, it is that many injuries can be prevented by proper conditioning, correct footwear, protective equipment (where appropriate) and a really thorough warm-up before play. However, even then, injuries do occur and, sooner or later you will be confronted with a decision as to whether you should treat yourself or enlist the aid of a doctor. Here are a few general rules:

Always call or see a doctor if:

- The incident causing the injury is a major one, such as a really severe fall in riding.
- The injury is on or near a joint or its associated ligaments.
- You are in severe pain.
- You have suffered unconsciousness, or feel a tingling or loss of sensation.
- You feel that the injury may be more severe or more complicated than you had first thought.

Also, if at any time an injury should:

- start to exude pus;
- show reddish streaks;
- start to show signs of swelling, or lead to swelling in the glands, especially those under the armpits or in the groin;
- or if you should begin to run a fever;

you should call a doctor *immediately*, as these are symptoms of infection.

Above all, call or see a doctor if any injury personally causes you concern. You won't be content until you have; and even if he can offer only reassurance, that is more than half the battle.

General Sports Ailments

Blisters

Blisters are probably the most frequent of all sports ailments and if not properly treated can develop into a painful (if temporary) handicap. They are particularly common at the start of the sporting season.

Blisters may appear wherever rubbing occurs, and the slightest discomfort caused by rubbing may very quickly result in a full-scale blister unless something is done about it.

The physical cause of a blister is the separation of layers of skin due to rubbing. This allows fluid, or occasionally blood—the blood blister—to collect between the layers. Continued rubbing eventually wears off the upper layer of skin, leaving a soft and potentially very painful underlayer of unhardened skin.

Treatment: A small blister can be contained by covering the affected area with a piece of adhesive tape. This ensures that the rubbing is against the tape rather than the skin.

A larger, more severe blister should first of all be cleansed with soap and water, or antiseptic. Next, sterilize a needle (either with antiseptic or in the flame of a match or cigarette lighter), allow it to cool, then carefully prick a hole at the edge of the blister. Gently press the top of the blister to drain the accumulated fluid or blood, but do not remove the protective skin. Keep dry and cover with an adhesive bandage. If the area remains painful or the pain increases, see a doctor.

Prevention: To avoid getting blisters on the feet, make sure that shoes fit properly, particularly at the sides and on top. Avoid shoes with internal stitching and high heel-tabs. New shoes should be broken in slowly, perhaps by wearing them around the house before using them in sport. Cotton socks absorb perspiration better than those made of artificial fibers.

Many runners and other sports enthusiasts coat their feet with vaseline to prevent rubbing; others prefer foot powder; and many perform with no socks at all—the solution is really whatever works best for you.

To harden the feet and the hands, dab them with alcohol or a skin-hardening agent. In some sports it is advisable to wear gloves at the beginning of the season until the hands harden.

Bruises

These are usually caused by a direct blow which breaks the small local blood vessels near the surface of the skin, causing a characteristic "black and blue" effect. Superficial symptoms of bruising and swelling may mask a deeper injury; if the blow causing the bruise was severe, it is advisable to have an X-ray.

Treatment: For minor bruises use what has come to be called the ICE (Ice, Compression, Elevation) treatment.

Ice: Apply directly, in an ice pack, in a plastic bag, or wrapped in a thin cloth—if ice is not available, run the injury under cold running water. This slows down the spread of the bruising and restricts swelling.

Compression: Cover or wrap the injured area with a bandage, compress or stretch bandage to keep down the swelling.

Elevation: If possible, raise the injured area above the level of the heart. This reduces the fluid pressure in the injured area.

Repeated courses of ICE treatment over 48 hours is usually enough to bring down the swelling, the first 6 hours after injury being the most important. If swelling persists or increases, it is usually best to see a doctor.

Cuts and Scrapes

Cuts and scrapes are as common on the sports field as they are off it, and they can occur in any sport. A cut or laceration is an actual tear in the skin that almost invariably results in bleeding; scrapes or abrasions are less deep and involve the removal of the outer layers of the skin.

Infection of cuts or scrapes can easily occur. Indications are an increase in pain in the injured area, which may also turn red and begin to swell. Puffiness and tenderness may also occur in the glands of the groin, armpits and neck. Temperature may rise. If any of these occur, see a doctor immediately; an antibiotic might be necessary.

Contamination of an open wound can result in tetanus. Many athletes guard against this by taking the precaution of having an antitetanus inoculation. (Make sure your antitetanus is up-to-date. A booster is needed every 10 years.)

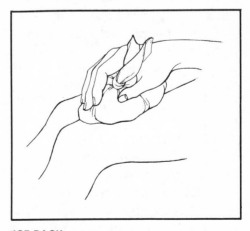

ICE PACK
Crush some ice and place in a cloth. Apply directly to site of bruise or injury.

To treat cuts: Stop the bleeding by applying a compress and keeping it in place for several minutes. Apply pressure with a clean finger if a compress is not available. Elevate the injured area, if possible, to help stop the bleeding. Then place the wound under cold running water, and clean it of all pieces of gravel, grit or dirt by gently dabbing it and the surrounding skin with antiseptic. You should then be able to see how deep the cut is.

If *shallow*, cover with an adhesive bandage.

If *deep*, with torn edges or if situated on a joint, a doctor must be consulted as suturing may be necessary.

To treat scrapes: Cleanse the wound as above. Next, examine the injured area. If the underlying skin layers appear whole, an application of antiseptic cream is usually sufficient. If possible, leave the injury open to the air to speed drying and healing. If the scrape is in a place where clothing may rub against it, a dry dressing of gauze and adhesive tape may be necessary.

If the underlying skin appears broken or in any other way damaged, consult a doctor; the injury may be more severe than first believed.

Burns

Burns as a result of falls are becoming increasingly common with the growing use of artificial surfaces. These are painful and can easily become infected.

Treatment: Apply cold water or ice to relieve immediate pain then thoroughly cleanse the wound. Cover with a dry, sterilized dressing.

Sunburn

Sunburn can be one of the most incapacitating of ailments in many sports. It is due to overlong exposure to the sun's ultraviolet rays, which burn off the outer layers of skin. By slowly conditioning the skin to the sun, burning is gradual, and most people slowly assume a tan (and with it, immunity to harmful rays). Sudden or prolonged exposure before the skin is ready, on the other hand, can cause severe sunburn. Sunburn susceptibility varies widely—fair-haired people are particularly vulnerable to burning.

Symptoms: Usually felt from 2–6 hours after exposure. Tenderness and redness, which in extreme cases can be agony to the touch. Occasionally blisters form and, as these dry, the dead layers of skin flake off (peeling).

Treatment: Apply cool water or a soothing ointment (most have a high oil content.) An oil/ice compress (1 part bath oil to 4 parts crushed ice, wrapped in a thin cloth) is also very soothing. Two aspirin (or substitute) every 4 hours also eases the discomfort.

Prevention: Common sense and awareness of the risks and likelihood of sunburn are the best preventatives. Certain environments and conditions render the risk higher: particularly the reflection of sun *on* water (affecting oarsmen, sailors, water skiers, surfers and windsurfers); and the effect of the sun *through* water (affecting swimmers and scuba divers). At higher altitudes, where the air is thin—even when there is some cloud cover—the effects of sunburn can be swift and savage. In winter at high altitudes where the air is dry and there is a strong sun, sunburn can be even more devastating.

To protect the skin: Sunscreen and sunburn preventative ointments are effective. Some can be bought which give a light tanning effect as well.

To protect the eyes: Sunglasses are essential (take a spare pair when skiing). Those with mirror lenses should be avoided, as they can reflect the sun on to the bridge of the nose.

Heat Exhaustion

Heat exhaustion is caused by loss of body water—dehydration—over a period of days. It is a gradual condition.

Symptoms: A fluctuating temperature and a pale, clammy skin. The victim is subject to prostration and collapse, appears weak and complains of headache and feeling tired, dizzy and shivery.

Treatment: Drink copious amounts of liquid, especially fruit juices.

Prevention: Avoid prolonged exposure to direct sunlight if possible, until fully acclimatized.

Heat Stroke or Sun Stroke

Unlike heat exhaustion, heat stroke can afflict suddenly and is potentially far more dangerous (sometimes lethal). It is caused by a total breakdown in the temperature control mechanism of the body. This can occur when the body is exposed to persistent high temperatures and/or a switch to high temperatures and high humidity, to which the body cannot acclimatize quickly enough. As a result, the temperature rises uncontrollably.

Symptoms: High temperature and a hot, dry skin. The victim complains of a burning sensation in lungs, muscles and legs. Breathing is difficult, painful and noisy. Headaches, blurred vision and feeling nauseous are common. The pulse pounds and the heat stroke sufferer may seem quite unaware of the surroundings, becoming confused and sometimes even delirious. Unconsciousness may follow.

Treatment: Speed is essential. Call for immediate medical attention, and while it is on the way lie the victim down in the shade with feet up. Remove clothing and pour quantities of water or any other liquid over the victim's body to help lower the body temperature. Ice, if available, is even better; water from a hose is also good.

Stop treatment when the victim appears to have recovered. Heat stroke may recur within an hour, so a constant watch must be kept. If it does recur, repeat treatment until proper medical assistance arrives.

After revival, large quantities of fruit juice should be drunk.

Frostbite

For those taking part in continuous exercise in winter (e.g., football and rugby players, skaters and cross-country skiers) the risks of frostbite are slight. It is those taking part in intermittent-exercise sports, such as downhill skiers (and beware those long cold periods in a ski lift), who are most in danger.

Frostbite occurs when the inner

layers of skin are literally destroyed by the freezing effect of cold weather. It is essential to take into account the wind as well as the cold here: the stronger the wind and the lower the outside temperature, the most chilling the effect. an outdoor temperature of 0°F and a 15 mph wind produces an effective temperature of −30°F, which is uncomfortably below the point at which exposed flesh will freeze within one minute.

Exposed areas, such as fingers, ears, nose and chin, are extremely susceptible to frostbite if not protected; also the toes, if boots are inadequately insulated.

Symptoms: The first symptom is a slight whitening of the exposed skin. This is caused by the blood vessels in the area "shutting off" and effectively cutting off the supply of blood to the tissues. This is accompanied by a feeling of cold and stiffness in the affected part.

Soon the whitened skin changes to a reddish color, as the body tries to compensate against the lowered temperature. The reddening is accompanied by a burning and stinging sensation, which soon develops into acute pain.

As the skin temperature drops, numbness sets in and the skin assumes a white waxy appearance.

Treatment: Immediate. If outdoors, make for shelter, especially from wind. Cover the frostbitten area with dry, gloved hands—*do not rub to try to get back the circulation.* Place frostbitten hands under the armpits. Give hot drinks if available.

As soon as possible rewarm the frost-bitten area in a warm-water bath at a temperature of 100–108°F, and *no hotter.* This should be done indoors or in a warm environment. Under no circumstances should the frostbitten part be allowed to refreeze.

Alcohol (brandy, etc.) is of only temporary benefit as a reviver. As it enlarges the blood vessels in the skin, its effect is actually to increase heat loss.

Prevention: Wear mittens with warm linings or inners; these are better than gloves as the fingers keep each other warm. Thick socks and well-insulated boots are essential; so is a warm woollen hat that can be pulled well down over the ears. A high collar is also advisable. Winter runners and cross-country skiers sometimes wear masks when facing into the wind; some cover their faces with vaseline before setting out.

Keep head and torso warm. In doubtful and cold weather when the possibilities of a sudden squall or shower are high, a light nylon or waterproof jacket, which can be folded into a pocket, is a useful precaution.

Exposure

Exposure occurs when the temperature of a body is lowered dramatically. First the skin loses heat, and this loss is transmitted to the deeper tissues and organs of the body. Exposure can be fatal if not recognized and treated immediately.

Causes: Accidental immersion in icy water, e.g., from a canoe or boat tipping over or ice giving way. A sudden icy rainstorm, which soaks an unprotected walker, runner or cross-country skier. Under both circumstances, wet clothes act as a conductor for the body's heat loss.

Symptoms: A visible slowing down of faculties. Speech becomes slow and slurred, vision distorted and the victim may begin to stumble. Increasing listlessness, light-headedness and possibly irritability with sudden changes of mood, as from laughter to tears, follows. The victim begins to shiver and may complain of cramps.

Treatment: Immediate *but gradual* rewarming is vital. Lie the victim down in shelter and out of the wind. Inactivity prevents further heat loss. If possible get two other people to lie down and cover the victim with their bodies. An even better method is to place the victim in a sleeping bag and get someone to climb in beside, having first removed wet clothing and wrapping the victim in dry clothes. Give sips of warm drinks, well laced with sugar. Do *not* use water bottles, etc.

Prevention: Be aware of the risks of winter exercise, especially in the mountains and away from habitation. Carry waterproof and warm clothing, and do not allow yourself to get wet in cold conditions.

When running or jogging in cold weather, it is advisable to plan your run so that you will go upwind on the way out and downwind on the way back.

MUSCLES, TENDONS AND LIGAMENTS

The MUSCLES generally control the movement of the limbs and every part of the body. TENDONS act as extensions to the muscles and anchor muscle to the bones of a joint. LIGAMENTS are fibrous straps which support and bind the bones together at the joints.

Muscle soreness

This is a very common sporting complaint and is due to overusing untuned muscles. It often occurs at the start of a season or after a long break, when the player is out of condition or when exercise changes suddenly in form or intensity.

Symptoms: Discomfort in the affected muscles which varies from mild stiffness to pain so intense that movement is almost impossible.

Treatment: Take a warm bath or shower and carry out gentle flexibility exercises (*see* Part I) while under water or while the muscles are still warm.

Prevention: Try to avoid sudden changes in type or intensity of exercise. Ease in gently to the anticipated new regime, especially at the start of the season.

Strains and Sprains

Strains and sprains are common in many sports, especially those which involve start-stop action or quick change of direction. They are usually due to an indirect injury such as a twist, turn or wrench, or because of general overstretching.

Sprains are partial tears to the ligament or tendon and usually occur at the ankle, knee, shoulder, thumb or finger. **Strains or pulls** may affect muscles, tendons or ligaments in such area as the back of the thigh (hamstring), ankle

(Achilles tendon), groin or elbow (as in tennis, golf or squash elbow).

Such injuries can take a long time to completely heal, and it is a mistake to attempt to return to sport too quickly.

Symptoms: A sudden, sharp and persistent pain at the site of the injury, often followed by swelling. If in the ankle, knee or hamstring, it is usually too painful to place weight on the injured leg.

Treatment: STOP before more injury is caused. Take the weight off the injured limb: wear a sling for the arm or use crutches in the case of a leg or ankle strain.

Rest. At the first opportunity apply ICE (see p. 225). After 48 hours try "contrast" treatments (hot and cold baths for 10 minutes at a time). If the pain is acute or accompanied by bruising, or if swelling persists for more than 24 hours, it is best to see a doctor. What you think is only a strain or sprain may turn out to be a fracture or dislocation.

Strains or sprains may take 2 weeks or more to heal—the older the person, the longer the healing time. Return to sport gradually and do not, on any account, hurry the process. As a muscle will shorten while healing, carry out stretching exercises when fit.

In the longer term, set about strengthening the muscles with appropriate exercises (*see* Part I).

Prevention: The best preventative is to have strong, well-toned and pliable muscles. Strains and sprains are often made more likely by inadequate warming-up, so warm up well before play. Many players in sports such as squash or tennis recommend that the warm-up should continue to the point of sweating.

Lack of flexibility is another important factor, so general conditioning should include stretching exercises, as in Part I. The hamstring pull is often due to an imbalance between the quadriceps muscles at the front of the upper leg and the usually less-exercised hamstrings at the back. Strengthening exercises should be designed to balance the relative power of the two.

Many strains and sprains are directly caused by wearing incorrect footwear. Using shoes with the proper studs, cleats or soles is essential. If the soles of your shoes are worn down, get new shoes. Shoes with high tops save many ankle injuries in start-stop sports. Taping of the ankle gives extra support to weak ankles or those athletes prone to ankle injuries.

Tendonitis (Tendinitis)

This is a common injury caused by the inflammation of a tendon within its tendon sheath (in which the tendon slides). Track athletes and those taking part in team and other running games are particularly subject to Achilles tendonitis. Those involved in throwing games—baseball, softball, cricket, rugby, field athletics—or players who use the smash shot, as in racquet sports, are apt to get tendonitis in the shoulder.

Symptoms: A nagging pain or great discomfort at the point of injury.

Treatment: On first feeling pain, stop all violent exercise; continuing play will aggravate the tendon and its associated sheath. If swelling develops, apply ICE (*see* p. 225); this will also lessen the pain. When the swelling and pain subsides, start *gradual* and *gentle* stretching exercises (*see* Part I). Heat treatments after 48 hours are also highly beneficial.

Prevention: If the condition persists or recurs, technique may be faulty (in which case consult a coach).

Muscle Spasms and Cramps

The exact cause of muscle spasms or cramps is still unknown, but it is believed that it could be due to an imbalance in the delicate chemical constitution of the muscle. This may occur as a result of dehydration in hot conditions.

Symptoms: Sudden and painful contractions of a muscle, which can last anywhere from a few seconds to several hours.

Treatment: Rubbing the affected area should help. In the case of thigh cramp, straighten the leg and, with the foot on the ground, press down on the knee. In the case of calf cramp, pinch the calf and at the same time bend the toes up as far as they will comfortably go; then work the ankle backward, forward and sideways.

If the cramp is sustained, deep massage and pummelling are also sometimes effective. The important thing is to try to stretch the cramped muscle.

Prevention: Although the quantity of salt in food is normally enough to keep the body supplied with sodium under ordinary circumstances, sprinkle on a little more in very hot weather or before energetic exercise in the heat. (Salt pills can have an adverse effect on the body and should not be taken.)

Stitch

The stitch is a form of muscle cramp in the upper abdomen and side. It is a common complaint especially with runners.

Symptoms: Sudden pain varying from slight and nagging to more severe and crippling. It usually subsides when exercise stops.

Treatment: Stop exercise altogether, if that is possible; otherwise slacken pace. Push the fingers into the side and bend forward. If that does not work, try bending sideways away from the cramp and sliding the hand as far down the leg as you can. When running, deep breaths may ease a stitch. Sips of warm water and gentle rubbing of the side and abdomen are usually effective in getting rid of a stitch.

Prevention: Avoid eating at all for at least 4 hours before energetic exercise. Before beginning to exercise, carry out stretching exercises for the abdomen (*see* Part I).

Specific Injuries and Conditions

EYES

Foreign Bodies

Pieces of grit, sand or dirt commonly find their way into the eye and can be very painful.

Treatment: Soak the eye in warm water to which a little salt has been added. An eye cup is the ideal container. Put the cup against the eye, tilt back your head, and blink the eye under the salty water. This should wash the foreign body to the corner, where it can be carefully removed with a clean handkerchief.

Black Eyes

Common in contact sports, black eyes are caused by direct contact with ball, stick or another player. If the vision is blurred or the pupils of the eyes are of different sizes, see a doctor immediately.

Treatment: Apply an ice pack or wet towel containing crushed ice over the eye for 15 minutes. Repeat periodically for 24–48 hours.

Prevention: The use of goggles and other eye protectors is becoming more frequent in some sports where eye injuries are quite common, such as in racquetball and squash.

For those wearing glasses, the risk of eye injury is higher. If glasses must be worn, ensure that they have sturdy rims and safety lenses. Tie them on with a piece of elastic or tape. Soft contact lenses are a good alternative, if you can wear them.

Lacerations of the Eyebrow

These are quite common in contact sports such as boxing, but by no means rare in other sports involving racquets, sticks or hard small balls.

Treatment: Apply cold sponge to prevent the eye from blackening. Then treat as for any other cut (*see* p. 226). If the wound is very close to the eye or there is any suggestion of vision being impaired, see a doctor immediately.

NOSE

Nosebleed

Treatment: Sit and lean forward over a basin. Spit out any blood; do not swallow it. Squeeze nose with thumb and forefinger for 3–6 minutes. Apply ice pack over nose. Ice at the back of the neck is also effective in helping to stop the bleeding. If bleeding continues, the nose may need packing by a doctor.

If the nose is broken, see a doctor.

SHOULDER
The shoulder is much used and is very vulnerable to injury in a variety of sports, especially throwing sports (baseball, football, cricket, bastketball and many field events in athletics) and sports that involve balancing (gymnastics, skating, etc.).

General overuse or sudden injury can cause fracture or dislocation. Wrenching can tear or strain associated muscles, tendons or ligaments.

Tendonitis (Tendinitis)
An overuse condition especially common in those sports where the arm is raised above the head—swimming, racquet games, throwing sports, etc.

Symptoms: Local pain, sometimes accompanied by swelling and bruising.

Treatment: Apply ice massage for the first 2 days. Rest from active sport is essential. Important, too, is to periodically move the shoulder gently; otherwise the condition may become aggravated and lead to "frozen shoulder." Carry out flexibility exercises (see Part I) as soon as the pain subsides. In addition, ice massage before exercise temporarily anesthetizes the shoulder and afterwards soothes the pain. After 48 hours, or when swelling has subsided, try heat treatments—e.g., hot towels, showers or baths. Aspirin (or suitable substitute) relieves inflammation.

If tendonitis recurs it may indicate incorrect technique. See a coach or professional for advice.

If pain persists for more than 2–3 weeks, steroid injections may be required. In any case it is best to see your doctor.

Prevention: Always warm up thoroughly before play and cool down afterwards. Carry out shoulder-strengthening exercises (see Part I) as part of your fitness routine.

Sprains and Strains
These can be due to falls or violent twists, or repeated small injuries. Lifting too heavy a weight is a common cause.

Treatment: As for other muscle problems, apply ice immediately. Keep shoulder in full motion as soon as possible. After 48 hours try contrast treatments of hot and cold baths, 10 minutes at a time. Carrying out shoulder-strengthening and flexibility exercises (see Part I) before the start of the season is advisable.

ARM
Tendonitis of the Biceps
The biceps muscles of the upper arm are liable to tendonitis, especially if subjected to sudden, unaccustomed use.

Symptoms: Tenderness or pain at the front of the upper arm, especially when flexed.

Treatment: Rest as much as possible. After 48 hours heat treatments give considerable relief.

ELBOW
Tennis Elbow (also Squash Elbow, Golf Elbow)

The causes of tennis elbow are many and varied, and by no means all associated with tennis. Anatomically, tennis elbow is inflammation of the attachments of the forearm muscles to the outer side of the elbow, aggravated by frequent shocks as the ball hits the racquet. Tennis elbow can occur in other racquet games (e.g., in squash—squash elbow), particularly where a wristy action is used; in Nordic (cross-country) skiing; in baseball as a result of throwing or pitching, and in other throwing sports, such as the javelin, hammer and shot put, or those where considerable weights are lifted, as in

MUSCLES OF THE FOREARM

Site of tennis elbow
Inflammation of the attachments of the forearm muscles to the outer side of the elbow.

Squash elbow is usually felt above the elbow joint.

Golfer's elbow is usually felt on the inside of the elbow joint.

weight lifting itself, wrestling and judo. It can also be aggravated by other less active pursuits, such as sawing wood or hammering, fly-fishing, hedge clipping, lifting buckets or suitcases, or at other times when the muscles are not geared up to undertake the task given them.

A similar complaint, golfer's elbow, is quite common with golfers. This tends to be caused by maintaining too tight a hand grip during the follow-through of the swing or in taking too big a divot out of the ground in an iron or chip shot.

Symptoms: A growing pain and tenderness. **Tennis elbow** is usually associated with pain on the outside of the elbow and the upper forearm, but this sometimes extends down toward the wrist; —it is extremely painful to extend the elbow fully. Occasionally, tennis elbow occurs on the inside of the elbow. At times the pain can also extend to the shoulder.

Golfer's elbow, on the other hand, is associated with pain on the inside of the elbow. Whereas **squash elbow** is normally felt just above the elbow.

Treatment: Tennis or squash elbow usually clears up after a few months, but this is providing total rest can be given. This not only precludes taking part in any sports which might aggravate the elbow but also means avoiding lifting any heavy weights in daily life—such as boxes, suitcases, buckets of water—or having your hand shaken too violently.

On first feeling tennis or squash elbow, it is advisable to stop playing immediately. Application of ice eases the discomfort. If very painful it could be worth putting your arm in a sling to lessen mobility of the elbow.

There are several other ways of alleviating tennis or squash elbow enough to be able to play. Many people use a brace or elasticized bandage placed at the top of the forearm below the elbow; others find a wrist strap more effective. In racquet sports, changing to a different size grip (or handle) may ease the pain. In tennis, using a racquet with a lighter head may also help. The racquet should not be strung too tightly as the tighter the stringing the greater the jarring effect when hitting the ball (50–54 pounds of tension is ideal). It is also believed that gut is kinder on the elbow than nylon.

Some tennis elbow sufferers advocate a thinner grip but most agree that a wider grip eases the pain more effectively (as do squash and badminton players). The handle must not be too large, however, or else it may lead to blisters on the playing hand and tired forearm muscles. Metal racquets have greater flexibility than wood racquets so switching to metal will take some of the jarring effect out of your shots.

There are many professional treatments for chronic tennis and squash elbow varying from injections to deep massage to immobilization in plaster.

Golfer's Elbow: Unlike tennis or squash elbow, golfer's elbow will not clear up of its own accord. Professional treatment is necessary, and this can include deep massage.

Gentle massage and kneading of the area while in a hot bath or shower will help to ease the pain. Alternatively, contrast hot and cold baths (10 minutes at a time) are beneficial. After play, immediate application of ice is also an effective means of easing discomfort.

Prevention (Tennis Elbow): Tennis elbow is principally due to incorrect stroking so the best way to prevent the condition is to use proper technique—and for this there is no substitute for correct coaching. A few general tips may be found under Tennis on pp. 132–133.

In general, stretching and strengthening exercises (Part I) should help to lessen the likelihood of these elbow injuries. The Broomstick Roll (S5) and the Tennis Ball Squeeze (S6) are particularly beneficial.

WRIST
Wrist injuries can be due to falls—such as in skiing, basketball, football, volleyball, racquet games and contact sports; or as a result of overstrain in such activities as weight lifting and some athletic field events; or as a result of incorrect hitting or batting technique in sports like baseball, softball and racquet games.

Wrist Sprain
Symptoms: Pain in the wrist, sometimes accompanied by swelling.

Treatment: ICE. This injury may mask a fracture, so it is important to have the wrist X-rayed as soon as possible. If no fracture is found, continue to keep the wrist moving. It may help to apply ice both before and after exercise.

HANDS
The hands are vulnerable to many injuries, particularly sprains and strains, often caused by awkward falls or catching a ball the wrong way, in combat sports, etc.

Strains and Sprains
Treatment: ICE. Maintain movement by opening and closing the fist.

Bruising
Often caused by direct contact with stick, ball, or other player. The bruising may well mask a fracture; if in any doubt, especially if the blow causing the fracture was very severe, it is best to have an X-ray.
Treatment: ICE. Maintain movement by exercises.

Mallet Finger (Baseball Finger)
Caused by the ball hitting the end of the fingers while attempting to catch it. Common in any ball game and extremely painful, it usually leads to swelling.
Treatment: ICE. Your doctor should splint the affected finger.

Tenosynovitis
Due to overuse and can be felt in the wrist, thumb or at base of fingers. In tennis or badminton constant overhead smashing can induce the condition in the wrist. Gymnasts, goalies and basketball, volleyball, handball and water polo players are prone to getting it in the thumb as well. In rowing, the condition is caused by gripping the oar too tightly.

Symptoms: Any movement of the wrist causes pain. There is often swelling at the wrist and base of the fingers.

Treatment: ICE. Maintain movement of the wrist and fingers.

Catching or Squeezing the Fingernails
This is quite common in sailing and water skiing.

Treatment: ICE.
Prevention: Keep fingernails short.

BACK
The back is very vulnerable to direct injuries, which usually result in bruising; and indirect injuries such as strains and sprains.

Bruising
Symptoms: Soreness, stiffness and sometimes swelling.

Treatment: ICE. After 48 hours, carry out contrast treatments of alternating hot and cold baths. Rest for 2–3 days.

Strains and Sprains
These are generally due to overuse, in particular violent stretching, and can occur in any sport where the arms are raised above the head—basketball, baseball, cricket, javelin throwing and other field events, tennis and other racquet sports. They are also common in sports involving lifting heavy weights—e.g., weight lifting, shot putting and hammer throwing—or those requiring violent body twists, such as high jumping.

Symptoms: Considerable muscle pain; loss of strength and some movement; sometimes visible bruising.

Treatment: Stop playing immediately. Apply ice to the back. It may be helpful to sleep on a bed board on the back, with a pillow under the knees for a few days. After 2–3 days start gentle flexibility exercises (*see* Part I), if not painful. Slow swimming is an excellent rehabilitation. Apply ice after exercise. Aspirin (or substitute) will ease the pain.

Prevention: Back strain is far less likely to occur with proper conditioning. Do strengthening and flexibility exercises (*see* Part I) before the start of the season.

Lower Back Pain
This is due to excessive stretching of the spinal ligaments and is often a consequence of lifting and bending. Weight lifters are frequent sufferers, as are squash and other ball game players who do a lot of low bending or stooping.

Symptoms: A sudden sharp pain in the lower back.

Treatment: Rest from sport. If the pain recurs, it is best to see a doctor. It may be helpful to sleep on a bed board on the back with a pillow under the knees for a few days.

Prevention: Adequate stretching and strengthening exercises (*see* Part I) before the start of the season.

Note: Lower back pain can mask a damaged disc. This is characterized by severe pain in the back that appears to reach down to the upper leg. Medical treatment is necessary.

CHEST
Winding
Shortness or loss of breath due to a blow in the *solar plexus,* a collection of nerves in the upper abdomen.

Treatment: Relax the muscles. Breathe in short and breathe out long. The sensation of not being able to breathe usually passes away in a few minutes.

Rib Stress Fractures
Due to overuse of the chest muscles; a common injury in tennis, rowing, weight lifting and gymnastics.

Symptoms: Chest pains, particularly on breathing out.

Treatment: Complete rest. If the pain persists see a doctor.

HIP
The hip is very vulnerable to bumps and bruises, especially in contact sports, skiing, skateboarding—due to falling on a hard surface—or colliding with another player or object.

Treatment: ICE. When swelling subsides, try contrast treatment of hot and cold baths. Avoid contact sports until fully healed. Try to keep weight off hip. Swimming is a useful interim sport.

THIGH
Hamstring Pull
The hamstring is situated at the back of the upper leg. Hamstring pulls are one of the most common sports injuries and can be completely incapacitating. They vary from mild to severe; even to complete rupture.

Cause: This is an overuse condition prompted by many different causes. In running it often occurs as the foot strikes the ground. In other sports it may be the result of the foot slipping, or the result of a faulty landing, such as in long or triple jumps on the athletic field.

Hamstring pulls are primarily due to an imbalance between the quadriceps muscles at the front of the upper leg and the hamstrings at the back, particularly in cases where the quadriceps have been overstretched at the expense of the hamstrings.

Symptoms: Pain, varying from mild to severe at the back of the leg—especially felt when sitting down—and may be felt all down the leg.

Treatment: ICE for 2–3 days and rest for 10–14 days, depending on severity. Taking aspirin or an equivalent is also helpful. Return gradually to sport after stretching exercises (*see* Part I) and then set about strengthening the hamstring muscles.

Prevention: Hamstring pulls are often due to overusing the muscle, before being fully ready. Tone up with preseason stretching and strengthening exercises before taking part in strenuous sport. Do not neglect the hamstrings when strengthening the quadriceps.

KNEE

The knee is particularly vulnerable to direct injuries from sticks or contact with other players, or indirect ones such as twists, sprains and wrenches.

Runner's Knee

Runner's knee is a collective term for a number of knee ailments primarily involving damage to the kneecap. It is common with runners—hence the name—but by no means uncommon in other sports, e.g., basketball knee.

Symptoms: Considerable pain just below and apparently behind the kneecap. This is particularly noticeable when running downhill or walking down slopes or stairs, because the angle of the knee irritates the kneecap when the foot strikes the ground. Sometimes a grating sensation can be felt. After rest the knee is decidedly stiff.

Treatment: The immediate remedy is to apply ice to relieve pain and discomfort. Cut down on all weight-bearing exercise and avoid hills wherever possible. In the long term if the discomfort persists, consult a foot specialist who may recommend orthotic foot supports, a knee brace and/or a special exercise program.

Prevention: Muscle-strengthening exercises lessen the chance of injury (*see* Part I). Arch supports and heel pads in the shoe which alter the angle of knee and leg when the foot hits the ground also help. Avoid downhill work early in the season.

Torn or Strained Knee Ligaments

These are especially common in contact sports and sports that involve start-stop action or quick turns. Skiers are especially vulnerable and artificial surfaces have led to an increase in knee injuries.

Symptoms: Tenderness, often severe pain after exercise, particularly when any weight is placed on the leg. Often swelling of the knee occurs.

Treatment: Apply ice to ease pain and reduce swelling. Rest for 2–3 days and then start *gentle* stretching exercises (*see* Part 1). In acute cases your doctor may decide to splint the knee.

Carry out knee-strengthening exercises when it is comfortable to do so (probably after 10 days). Until the knee is strong again, strapping during the day is advisable.

Prevention: Proper early-season conditioning is the best preventative. Use correct studs or cleats, according to the playing surface.

SHIN
Shin Splints

A condition arising from the overuse of the muscle fibers of the shin, which pull away from the bone, resulting in inflamed muscles and tendons. It is commonly caused by running on hard, unyielding surfaces, especially by undertrained athletes at the start of the season. Runners and football and basketball players are particularly vulnerable.

Symptoms: First indication is a tightness in the lower leg, especially after heavy exercise. The more you exercise, the more evident the tightness, which does not go away during rest. Also pain can often be felt down the front and side of the leg.

Treatment: Applying ice after exercise usually eases the discomfort considerably. A change to a well-padded

and flexible shoe or using spongy innersoles also eases the pain. Until the condition is better, exercise gently and gradually, and always on soft surfaces. Exercises to strengthen the leg muscles (*see* Part I) should be carried out as soon as comfortable. Swimming and bicycling are good rehabilitation activities.

Prevention: *See under* Stress Fractures *below.*

Stress Fractures

These are microscopic cracks in the bone, which at first do not show up on an X-ray. They are brought about by continuous jolting and jarring, and are particularly common in long-distance runners, road runners and race walkers, although other athletes are by no means immune. Stress fractures most commonly occur in the bones of

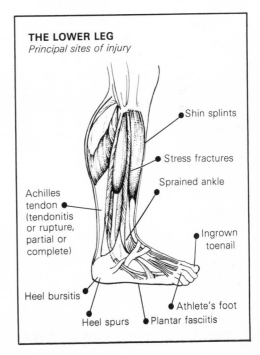

THE LOWER LEG
Principal sites of injury

Shin splints

Stress fractures

Sprained ankle

Achilles tendon (tendonitis or rupture, partial or complete)

Ingrown toenail

Heel bursitis

Athlete's foot

Heel spurs

Plantar fasciitis

the leg, but they may also occur in the feet and hands.

Symptoms: After a period of activity a throbbing pain is felt deep in the shin. This increases if running or other training is continued at the same intensity.

Treatment: Rest or reduced activity usually alleviates the condition. Ice massage gives considerable local relief. Temporarily take up another sport and return to full activity in your own sport slowly and gradually. Discomfort may be eased by taping or strapping. An extra heel sole may also be helpful.

Prevention (for both Shin Splints and Stress Fractures): Both conditions are associated with early-season activity and undertrained athletes. Thus a general-conditioning and strengthening course is desirable.

Use common sense in not exercising on surfaces that are too hard, especially at the start of the season and before being fully conditioned. Wear good, flexible shoes with soft innersoles to prevent jarring unconditioned feet.

ANKLE
Ankle Sprain
Common on and off the sports field. Either due to the ankle turning inward—during walking, running or jumping—or when the ankle turns outward as usually happens in falling.

Symptoms: A sharp pain in the ankle area, so sharp in most cases that it is almost impossible to place any weight on the injured foot.

Treatment: ICE and rest. If after the ice treatment you are unable to walk as before, see a doctor; the sprain may be more severe than you at first thought, but bear in mind that ankle sprains always seem worse the second day. Rest for several days to give the sprain time to recover. Then carry out gentle stretching exercises (*see* Part I).

Prevention: Many sprained ankles are due to carelessness. Try to avoid uneven surfaces, rough grass or slippery ground. Good footwear is essential, and shoes designed for weak ankles are now made. Exercise to strengthen the ankles (*see* Part I) and ankle taping will give additional support.

ACHILLES TENDON
The Achilles tendon is the broad muscular strap which runs down the back of the calf to the heel. It is peculiarly vulnerable to overuse injuries. Inflammation or more severe conditions of the Achilles tendon are some of the most frequent ailments affecting athletes.

Achilles Tendonitis (Tendinitis)
This is a condition brought about by overexercising the ankle, especially if it is neither strong enough nor pliable enough to stand strain. As a result, the tendon becomes swollen and inflamed. This results in pain varying from mild to acute.

Treatment: Rest is the best treatment, but many athletes prefer to carry on and rely on other methods. These often involve the use of ice immediately after exercise. An extra heel or heel cup inside the shoe alters the tilt of the ankle and prevents the tendon from becoming overstretched, giving considerable relief.

Until the condition is improved do not overuse the foot. Avoid uphill work or exercising on hard or rough surfaces. This is not only extremely painful, it could make the condition worse and lead to a partially ruptured or ruptured Achilles tendon, where the tendon actually snaps. If this occurs an operation may be necessary. Total rest is essential in any case.

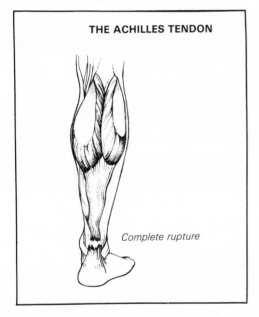

THE ACHILLES TENDON

Complete rupture

FOOT
Athlete's Foot

A condition caused by a variety of fungi that thrive in damp or wet conditions. The spores are picked up in shower areas or around the edges of swimming and plunge pools.

Some people are more susceptible to athlete's foot than others. The most likely areas of infection are beneath the foot and between the toes—particularly the third, fourth and fifth toes.

Symptoms: Athlete's foot is accompanied by a burning, itching sensation, which is worsened by scratching. Often a damp white fungus shows on the infected areas, or a mild rash which at times gives off a yeast-like smell.

Treatment: Athlete's foot can usually be cleared up by using antifungal powder, which is easily obtainable. If there is no improvement within two weeks consult a doctor, as apparent athlete's foot can disguise other skin ailments.

Prevention: Keep the foot as dry as possible, particularly between the toes. After showering, dry them throughly and apply powder, again particularly between the toes. Change socks frequently and make sure they are thoroughly washed. Use talcum or other foot powder inside shoes.

Plantar Fasciitis

Symptoms: A dull aching pain in the sole of the foot in the region of the heel. In extreme form it can lead to swelling.

Cause: Strain, tear or occasionally rupture of the *plantar fascia,* the tissue stretching across the sole of the foot from the heel to the ball. The injury can be due to a number of causes: a sudden turn of the foot; shoes without proper arch support or soles which are too stiff; feet which roll inward too much when walking.

Occurs commonly with skiers, both alpine and Nordic, due to lacing or buckling boots too tightly; gymnasts, who are inclined to land on the ball of the foot; fast bowlers in cricket; hurdlers; long jumpers; etc.

Treatment: The only satisfactory treatment is resting the foot and not placing any weight on it. To reduce swelling, apply ice. Pads and taping give additional support and ease the pain. Return to sport gradually and continue the ice treatment until all pain has ceased.

Prevention: Using orthotic devices to support the arch of the foot or heel wedges to adjust the tilt of the heel is effective in many cases. Persistent sufferers should seek the advice of a foot specialist.

Heel Spurs
This is a condition closely allied with plantar fasciitis (*see above*).

Symptoms: Considerable pain when any weight is placed on the heel.

Cause: Abnormal strain on the *plantar fascia* where it attaches to the underside of the heel bone. With constant irritation a small protrusion or spur of bone develops.

Treatment: To reduce pain and swelling, apply ice as in plantar fasciitis. Heel padding is highly successful in the treatment of this condition; the use of horseshoe-shaped inner heels takes all the weight off the painful part of the heel.

Prevention: *See* plantar fasciitis *above*.

Heel Bursitis
This condition can be closely linked with plantar fasciitis and heel spurs (*see above*). Constant irritation in the heel area causes the heel bursae to become inflamed and swollen. (A bursa is a small sac of fluid which acts as a lubricated surface and shock absorber in the joint.)

Symptoms and **treatment** are the same as for plantar fasciitis and heel spurs. If the pain does not subside after a week, consult a foot specialist.

A more common form involves the bursae between the heel bone and the Achilles tendon running down the back of the heel.

It is associated with a feeling of a deep "blister," a tenderness and spongy sensation at the back of the heel. Apply ice to reduce swelling and help the discomfort, and use padding—in this case thin, as it must fit between the heel of the foot and the back of the shoe. Orthotic devices as recommended by a specialist can do much to help both forms of heel bursitis.

TOENAILS
Ingrown Toenail
Athletes should trim their toenails frequently, making sure that the ends of the nails are cut square. Failure to do this can result in a situation in which the constant banging and pressing of the toes against the end of the shoe (especially if the shoe is too narrow at the toe end) forces the toenail into the soft flesh at the side of the toe. This can be extremely painful and lead to infection. It is eased by padding, but it is advisable to have a doctor trim the side of the nail.

Blackened Toenail (Runner's Toenail)

Occasionally a blood clot forms beneath the nail. This can be a very painful condition.

Treatment: Unbend a paperclip, or take a needle and heat it in the flame of a match or cigarette lighter until red hot. Then carefully burn a hole through the nail to allow the accumulated blood to escape. Wash the foot well before and after treatment; apply a dry dressing.

First Aid for the Sports Field

Insect Stings
Remove the sting with tweezers or the point of a needle sterilized in the flame of a match or lighter. Apply a recommended cream, ice or failing that, a cold compress—this reduces discomfort and swelling. If the sting is in the mouth (particularly in the tongue or gums) where swelling might block the air passage, call a doctor immediately. In the meantime give the victim ice to suck.

Dog Bites
Wash the animal's saliva away from the wound. Cleanse the wound thoroughly with soap and water, and cover with a dry bandage. If severe, or in a country where rabies might be present, call a doctor immediately.

Bleeding (External)
Heavy bleeding must be stopped immediately. Press directly on the wound, if necessary holding the edges together by hand until a bandage is available. It may be necessary to maintain pressure for anything from 5 to 15 minutes.

When possible, and while still maintaining pressure on the wound, sit or lie the victim down. Raise the bleeding part, if possible, above the level of the heart—unless a fracture is suspected. Apply a large dressing. If blood soaks through this, apply further dressings. Call a doctor as soon as you can.

Dislocations
Dislocations of a joint are caused by a severe twist, turn or wrench—this displaces the joint itself and tears the ligaments supporting it. Dislocations of the shoulder, elbow, thumb, fingers and jaw are especially common.

Symptoms: Extreme pain and inability to move the joint. The joint itself is distorted and swollen, and there is occasionally numbness in the limb. An apparent dislocation may also mask a fracture.

Treatment: Move the limb as little as possible and make no attempt to put the joint back in place. Call a doctor. Meanwhile support the limb in the most comfortable position, using padding, a sling or bandages as necessary.

Displaced Cartilage of the Knee

Caused by a direct blow or a sudden wrench—as when missing a kick in football, or in slipping when the leg is twisted. The most usual cause is a twist or side blow given to a weight-bearing leg—as when running to retrieve a ball, or reaching for a wide shot in racquet sports.

Symptoms: Severe pain, especially on the inner side of the knee. The knee is bent and cannot be straightened and any attempt to do so leads to more pain. There is tenderness over the displaced cartilage and often swelling at the site of injury.

Treatment: See a doctor. This is an injury which must be treated professionally at the outset. In the meantime, raise and support the leg. Protect the knee with any padding you can find, and hold it in place with a bandage. Cartilage trouble often recurs. Sometimes an operation to remove the cartilage may become necessary.

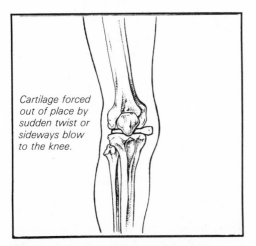

Cartilage forced out of place by sudden twist or sideways blow to the knee.

DISPLACED CARTILAGE OF THE KNEE

Fainting

This is caused by a sudden lowering of blood pressure which results in a temporary reduction of the flow of blood to the brain. It may be triggered by any number of causes, but the most usual is excessive heat, particularly in a confined space. It also frequently occurs as a result of shock following a severe injury involving heavy bleeding or bruising, burns, fracture or dislocation or after a major fall.

Indications that fainting is about to occur: Loss of color; clammy or sweaty skin. The victim may start to yawn or sway and appear giddy or dizzy. The pulse is weak but rapid. Breathing is quick and shallow, sometimes gasping. A person about to faint usually complains of feeling nauseous, and is sometimes very thirsty.

Prevention: If you suspect that someone is about to faint, urge the victim to breathe deeply and lie down in the shade. Raise the feet above the level of the heart. Loosen tight clothing. Cover with a coat to keep warm. Do not leave unattended.

On loss of consciousness, call for a doctor. Meanwhile move the victim as little as possible, but place in shade if close at hand. Raise the feet above the level of the heart. Turn head to one side. Loosen tight clothing. Again do not leave the victim unattended. If breathing is difficult, place in the

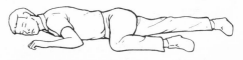

RECOVERY POSITION

245

recovery position (*see* p. 245). As the victim recovers, raise to a sitting position.

FRACTURES

The most common fractures in sport are to the arm, leg, collarbone, ribs, jaw, skull and occasionally to the spine or neck. These are almost always due to either a direct blow—from stick, ball or opponent—or as a result of a violent twist or awkward fall.

General Treatment: Call a doctor immediately. Move the injured person as little as possible. The severity of the incident may give some indication of the seriousness of the injury.

The injured person may also be suffering from shock (for treatment, *see* Fainting: On Loss of Consciousness *above*).

Broken Limbs

Symptoms: Severe pain and extreme tenderness at the site of injury, accompanied by swelling and bruising. The injured person is unable to move the limb, and the bone may be seen to be clearly distorted. Sometimes the bone breaks through the skin.

Treatment: If the victim has to be moved, support the broken limb in the most comfortable position. Use a sling for an arm, wrist or finger fracture to prevent jarring.

In the event of a broken leg, place the injured person on any solid platform—a plank, door, shutter, etc.—and when moving take the greatest care. It is usually best to strap down the victim using

bandages or any other ties that may be available. To prevent movement of the injured leg, use a splint to maintain rigidity; this can be a stick, pole or even the victim's uninjured leg. Straps and ties must be tight enough to prevent movement, but not so tight as to cut off circulation. Check every 10 minutes to see that swelling beneath the strappings will not cause discomfort.

Broken Collarbone (Clavicle)

Symptoms: The site of the injury is very painful and usually accompanied by swelling. The bone is seen to be severely distorted and the arm on the injured side is partially helpless.

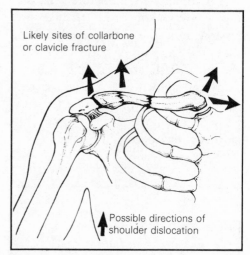

Likely sites of collarbone or clavicle fracture

Possible directions of shoulder dislocation

SHOULDER INJURIES
A fall on an outstretched hand or direct fall on the shoulder may cause a broken clavicle or collarbone, or lead to a dislocated shoulder.

Treatment: Until medical help is available, support the arm on the broken side with a sling to prevent jarring.

Broken Ribs

A severe blow can drive the broken

ends into a lung, which can be an extremely dangerous condition. All rib fractures should be seen as soon as possible by a doctor.

Symptoms: Sharp pain at the site of the injury which is made worse when the victim breathes deeply. As a result the injured person usually takes short, shallow breathes.

Treatment: Support the arm on the fractured side in a sling to prevent jarring and discomfort.

Broken Jaw

This is usually the result of a direct blow to the jaw, as in boxing or in stick games.

Symptoms: Pronounced distortion of the jaw. The jaw is extremely painful, especially when talking or swallowing.

Treatment: Support the jaw with the hand or a soft bandage bound to the top of the head while awaiting medical attention. If the injured person wants to vomit, turn the head to one side and support the jaw. Remove false teeth.

Fractured Skull

This calls for *immediate* medical assistance. *Do not move the victim.*

Symptoms: Blood or straw-colored liquid may come from the ear or the nose. The eyes may appear bloodshot, and may later blacken. Severe bruising or swelling appears on the head.

Treatment: Lay the injured person in the recovery position while awaiting medical help. Should the victim stop breathing, carry out immediate artifi-

cial respiration (*see* Resuscitation, pp. 248–250).

Fractured Spine

This calls for *immediate* medical attention. *Do not move the victim at all,* if possible. Incorrect treatment can lead to permanent damage to the spinal column and paralysis of the limbs.

Symptoms: Severe pain in the back. Possible loss of power and sensation in the limbs.

Treatment: It is vital that the injured person stay as still as possible to prevent damage to the spinal cord.

On land: tell the injured person to lie absolutely still until medical help arrives. Cover with a blanket or coat to keep warm.

In the water (after a diving, boating or surfing accident): Keep the victim's head above water to prevent drowning. It is essential to keep the spine and head in an absolutely straight line; if the head or neck bend, the spinal column is likely to be damaged. Ease the victim on to a solid board. The best way to do this is with a four-man lift—one at the head, one at the feet and one on each side. Many pools and swimming areas have spinal boards or a stretcher which can be immersed in the water. Failing these, any board or plank will have to suffice. Having eased the victim on to his back on the board, prevent the head turning by placing blankets or clothes on either side. Then very slowly and carefully bring the victim ashore.

Concussion

Concussion is sometimes called (and is

equivalent to) "brain shaking." It can be caused by a fall on the head, a heavy blow to the jaw or even being knocked down hard into a sitting position. Concussion should always be suspected after a heavy fall, particularly in riding. It is not necessarily followed by unconsciousness. A doctor should always be consulted.

Symptoms: In most cases, partial or complete loss of consciousness for a brief period. The face may be pale, the skin cold and clammy, the pulse rapid and faint. There may be weakness, even temporary paralysis of the limbs. The victim may show irritability, confusion, disorientation and other uncharacteristic behavior.

Treatment: Call a doctor *immediately*. If the victim is unconscious and has stopped breathing, start artificial respiration without delay (*see below*). Otherwise place in the recovery position in shade. Loosen clothing at neck and waist.

The condition of **compression**, when there is actual pressure on some part of the brain, may take place sometime after the injury. This is highly dangerous and *immediate* medical attention is vital.

Symptoms: Increasing drowsiness and a dilation of one or both pupils of the eye. The injured person's breathing may become noisy, the body temperature may rise.

RESUSCITATION
(ARTIFICIAL RESPIRATION)
If an injured person loses consciousness and stops breathing, resuscitation *must*

begin at once. Every second is vital. In the case of a water accident, begin treatment as soon as the head is out of the water.

There are two principal methods of resuscitation involving artificial respiration: **mouth-to-mouth** (or **mouth-to-nose**), when air from the rescuer's lungs is breathed into those of the victim; and the **Holger Nielsen method**, which is used when facial injuries make the use of the mouth-to-mouth method impossible (this involves moving the victim's arms and chest to make the lungs expand and contract). In addition, **heart compression** must be used when the heart has stopped beating.

Mouth-to-Mouth
First remove anything likely to block the air passage from the mouth. (Check for false teeth and, if necessary, clean the mouth of vomit or other debris.) Then tilt the head back until it is possible to see down the nostrils (*a*). Pinch the nostrils between finger and thumb to seal the nose air passage and to ensure that when you breathe into the victim's mouth no air escapes from the nose.

With the fingers and thumb of the other hand press forward the lower jaw so that the chin juts forward. This opens the mouth and lifts the tongue clear of the airway.

Take a deep breath, open your mouth wide and place your lips around those of the victim (*b*). Blow firmly but gently into the victim's mouth. (Out of the corner of your eye look at the victim's chest, which should expand.)

Lift off your mouth to get another

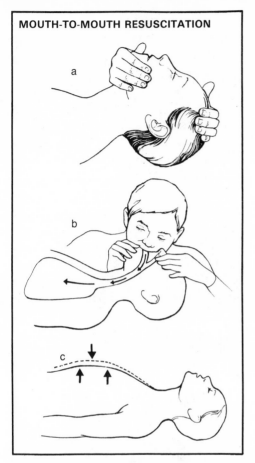

MOUTH-TO-MOUTH RESUSCITATION

a

b

c

breath. (The victim's chest should then clearly be seen to fall as the air is expelled—*c*).

Continue treatment at a steady rate of 10 breaths per minute (1 every count of 6). The proof that your treatment is working is the steady rise and fall of the victim's chest. When colour comes back into the victim's face and natural breathing starts again, you may stop. But it is still important to keep a close watch on the victim as the treatment may need to be repeated.

When carrying out mouth-to-mouth resuscitation on a child, it will

probably be easier to place your mouth over both the nose and mouth. Use much less force in blowing air into a child's lungs than into an adult's.

In the event of an injury to the mouth or jaw, the **mouth-to-nose** method should be used. Keep the victim's mouth shut while carrying out the treatment. It is important, however, to keep the jaw forward.

Holger Nielsen

This is used when facial injuries make mouth-to-mouth or mouth-to-nose resuscitation impracticable.

Place the victim on his front, with arms forward and head to one side and resting on the hands (*see* illustrations, p. 250).

Position yourself on one knee close to the victim's forehead, with the foot of the other leg near his elbow (*a*).

Place the hands, with fingers splayed out and thumbs touching, on the victim's back on a line from armpit to armpit. Rock forward, pressing down on the victim's back until your arms are nearly vertical (*b*). This pressure on the victim's chest will empty lungs.

Rock backwards and slip your hands to the victim's armpits and down the arms to just above the elbow (*c*). At the same time raise the injured person's elbows, pulling them toward you slightly, until you feel resistance (*d*). This has the effect of expanding the chest and filling the lungs.

Let the elbows fall back and repeat the alternate back pressing and elbow raising. The cycle should last about 6 seconds and be smooth and rhythmical.

THE HOLGER NIELSEN METHOD OF ARTIFICAL RESPIRATION

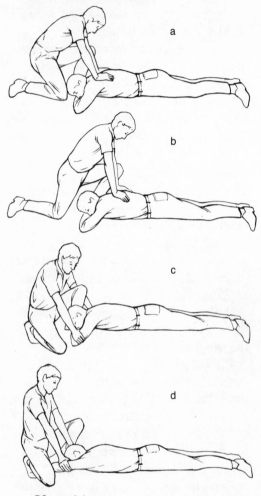

If vomiting occurs at any time, make sure the mouth is cleared before you continue.

The steady rocking movement should provide all the pressure needed; do not force down on the back. Apply much less force if victim is a child.

When the victim starts to breathe again normally, place in the recovery position (*see* p. 245). Keep a close watch in case breathing stops again.

Heart Compression

Should there be no sign of response in the victim after 4 movements of the chest during artificial respiration, then the heart has probably stopped beating. It is vital to get it started again.

Tap the chest smartly once over the lower part of the breastbone. If this does not start the heart beating again, then use the following procedure.

Kneel alongside the victim. Place the heel of one hand on the lower part of the breastbone (*see* illustration), keeping the palms and fingers clear of the chest. Then with arms straight, rock forward, pressing down the lower part of the victim's breastbone. Then relax arms.

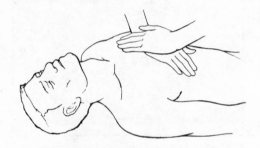

Carry out this movement quickly: 60 times a minute for adults; 80 times a minute for children.

Signs of response are a renewed beat of the heart and a return of natural color.

If alone: Carry out a cycle of 2 inflation of the lungs by mouth-to-mouth resuscitation followed quickly by 15 heart compressions.

If you have help: One person should carry out mouth-to-mouth resuscitation while the other performs the heart compression. Do so at a rate of 2 inflations to 5 heart compressions.

Bibliography

I. GENERAL REFERENCES

GENERAL FITNESS AND CONDITIONING

Astrand, Dr. Per-Olof. *Health and Happiness.* New York: Barron's/Woodbury, 1977.

Diagram Group, The. *The Complete Encyclopedia of Exercises.* New York and London: Paddington Press, 1979.

The Fitness Challenge in the Later Years. New York: US Government Printing Office, 1973.

Higdon, Hal. Fitness after Forty. Mountain View, Ca: World Publications, 1977.

An Introduction to Physical Fitness and Sports. New York: US Government Printing Office, 1976.

Man, John. *Walk.* New York and London: Paddington Press, 1979.

Morehouse, Laurence E., and Gross, Leonard. *Total Fitness in 30 Minutes a Week.* London: Mayflower Books, 1977.

Rose, Kenneth, and Martin, Jack Dies. *The Lazy Man's Guide to Physical Fitness.* Totowa, NJ: Condor, 1977.

Royal Canadian Air Force. *Exercise Plans for Physical Fitness.* New York: Simon and Schuster, 1962.

Tulloh, Bruce. *Natural Fitness.* New York: Simon and Schuster, 1976. London: Arrow Books, 1978.

Stewart, Pat, ed. *US Fitness Book.* New York: Simon and Schuster, 1979.

DIET

Atkins, Dr. Robert C. *Diet Revolution.* New York: Bantam Books, 1974.

Gelb, Barbara Levine. *The Dictionary of Food.* New York and London: Paddington Press, 1978.

Kraus, Barbara. *Calories and Carbohydrates.* New York: Signet Books, 1975.

Manley, Derek. *Diet Book for Diet Haters.* London: Corgi, 1976.

Mayer, Jean. *Diet for Living.* New York; McKay, 1975.

Milo, Mary. *Diet and Exercise Guide.* New York: Arno, 1976.

Palm, Daniel. *Diet away Your Stress, Tension and Anxiety.* New York: PB, 1977.

SPORTS MEDICINE

Colson, John H. C., and Armour, William J. *Sports Injuries and Their Treatment.* London: Stanley Paul, 1979.

Fahey, Thomas D. *What to Do about Athletic Injuries.* New York: Butterick Publishing, 1979.

Key, James D. *The Week-End Athlete's Guide to Sports Medicine.* Winter Park, FLA: Anna Publishing Inc., 1979.

Mirkin, Dr. Gabe, and Hoffman, Marshall. *The Sportsmedicine Book.* Boston: Little, Brown, 1978.

Muckle, David S. *Sports Injuries.* London: Oriel Press, 1977.

Sheehan, Dr. George. *The Encyclopedia of Athletic Medicine.* Mountain View, CA: World Publications, 1977.

The Sunday Times Book of Body Maintenance. London: Michael Joseph, 1978.

Tucker, W. E., and Castle, Molly. *Sportsmen and Their Injuries.* London: Pelham Books, 1978.

II. SPORT BY SPORT (ALPHABETICAL ORDER)

AIKIDO

Tohei, Koichi. *A Coordination of Mind and Body for Self-Defense.* London: Souvenir Press, 1966.

Tohei, Koichi. *This Is Aikido.* London: Japan Publications, Inc., 1975.

Yamada, Yoshimitsu. *Aikido Complete.* New York: Citadel Press, 1974.

ARCHERY

Heath, E. G. *The Art of Archery.* London: Kaye and Ward, 1978.

Heath, E. G. *Archery, the Modern Approach.* London: Faber and Faber, 1978.

McKinney, Wayne C. *Archery.* Dubuque, Ia: William C. Brown, 1975.

ATHLETICS—see under TRACK AND FIELD

BADMINTON

Davis, Pat. *Badminton Complete*. London: Kaye and Ward, 1975.

Mills, Roger. *Badminton*. Wakefield, Yorkshire: E. P., 1978.

Mills, Roger, and Butler, Eric. *Tackle Badminton*. London: Stanley Paul, 1977.

BASEBALL AND SOFTBALL

Bethell, Dell. *The Complete Book of Baseball Instruction*. Chicago: Contemporary Books, 1978.

Groch, Dick. *Mastering Baseball*. Chicago: Contemporary Books 1978.

Harrelson, Bud. *How to Play Better Baseball*. New York: Atheneum, 1972.

Soderholm, Eric. *Conditioning for Baseball*. Winter Park, FLA: Anna Publishing Inc., 1978.

Joyce, Joan and Anguillare, John, *Winning Softball*. Chicago: Contemporary Books, 1975.

Spackman, Robert R., Jr. *Conditioning for Baseball*. Springfield ILL: C. C. Thomas, 1967.

BASKETBALL

Coleman, Brian E. *Basketball Techniques, Teaching and Training*. Cranbury, NJ: A. S. Barnes, 1978. London: Kaye and Ward, 1975.

Goodrich, Gail. *Winning Basketball*. Chicago: Contemporary Books, 1976.

Naysmith, Brian and Hill, Terry. *Basketball*. Newton Abbot, Devon: David and Charles, 1978.

BOXING

Fleischer, Nat. *Training for Boxers*. Bridgeport, CT: Impress House, 1977.

James, David. *Better Boxing*. New York: Soccer, 1978. London: Kaye and Ward, 1977.

Schroeder, Charles E. *Boxing Skills for Fun and Fitness*. New York: Ragmar Publications, 1973.

CANOEING

Angier, Bradford and Taylor, Zack. *Introduction to Canoeing*. Harrisburg, PA: Stackpole, 1973.

Bridge, Raymond. *The Complete Canoeist's Guide*. New York: Scribner, 1978.

Bridge, Raymond. *The Complete Guide to Kayaking*. New York: Scribner, 1978.

Ruck, Wolfgang E. *Canoeing and Kayaking*. New York: McGraw Books, 1976.

CRICKET

Illingworth, Ray. *Spin Bowling*. London: Pelham Books, 1978.

The M.C.C. *Cricket Coaching Book*. London: Heinemann, 1976.

Willis, Bob. *Pace Bowling*. London: Pelham Books, 1978.

CYCLING

Luther, Kenneth E. *Bicycling for Fun and Good Health*. Hollywood, CA: Wilshire, 1977.

Woodland, Les. *Cycle Racing and Touring*. New York: Transatlantic Publications, 1977.

Woodland, Les. *Better Competitive Cycling*. London: Kaye and Ward, 1978.

DIVING

Armbruster, David A. *Swimming and Diving*. New York: Mosley, 1973.

Rackham, George. *Diving Complete*. London: Faber and Faber, 1975.

FENCING

Anderson, Bob. *Better Fencing*. London: Kaye and Ward, 1973.

Lownds, Camille and August, Tony. *Foil Around and Stay Fit*. New York: Harcourt Brace Jovanovich, 1977.

Manley, Albert. *Complete Fencing*. New York: Doubleday, 1978.

FOOTBALL

Conklin, Mike. *Inside Football*. Chicago: Contemporary Books, 1978.

Darden, Ellington. *Conditioning for Football*. Winter Park, FLA: Anna Publishing Inc., 1979.

Olson, O. Charles. *Prevention of Football Injuries*. Philadelphia, PA: Lea and Febiger, 1971.

GOLF

Alliss, Peter and Trevillion, Paul. *Easier Golf*. London: Stanley Paul, 1978.

Jennison, Keith, and Pratt, William A. *Year-Round Conditioning for Part-Time Golfers*. New York: Atheneum, 1978.

Snead, Sam and Aultman, Dick. *Golf Begins at Forty*. New York: Dial, 1978.

GYMNASTICS

Prestidge, Pauline. *Women's Gymnastics for Performer and Coach*. London: Faber and Faber, 1975.

Spackman, Robert R., Jr. *Conditioning for Gymnastics*. Springfield, ILL: C. C. Thomas, 1970.

Stuart, Nik. *Gymnastics for Men*. London: Stanley Paul, 1978.

HANDBALL (COURT)

Reznik, John W. *Championship Handball by the Experts*. New York: Leisure Press, 1976.

Yessis, Michael. *Handball*. Dubuque: William C. Brown, 1977.

HANDBALL (TEAM)

Aagard, Talle. *Mini Handball*. Roaskilde (Denmark), 1978.

ABC Illustrated Coaching Textbook. International Handball Federation, 1978.

HOCKEY, FIELD

Clarke, Trevor. *Teaching and Playing Hockey*. London: Lepus Books, 1976.

Flint, Rachel H. *Field Hockey*. New York: Barron, 1978.

Hockey Coaching. London, The Hockey Association: Hodder and Stoughton, 1975.

HOCKEY, ICE

Fullerton, James H. *Ice Hockey, Playing and Coaching*. New York: Hastings, 1978.

Hayes, Don. *Ice Hockey* (Physical Education Series). Dubuque, Iowa: William C. Brown, 1972.

JOGGING AND RUNNING

Fixx, James F. *The Complete Book of Running*. New York: Random House, 1977.

Geline, Robert. *The Practical Runner*. New York: Collier Books, 1978.

Henderson, Jow. *Jog, Run and Race*. Mountain View, CA: World Publications, 1977.

Hewitt, James. *Jogging Your Way to Health and Fitness*. London: New English Library, 1978.

Sheehan, Dr. George. *Doctor Sheehan on Running*. New York: Bantam Books, 1975.

Temple, Cliff. *Jogging for Fitness and Pleasure*. New York: Worlds Work, 1977.

JUDO

Frommer, Harvey. *The Martial Arts: Judo and Karate*. New York: Atheneum, 1978.

Tegner, Bruce. *Judo Sport Technique for Physical Fitness and Tournament*. Ventura, CA: Thor, 1976.

Tegner, Bruce. *Karate and Judo Exercises: Physical Conditioning for the Oriental Sport Fighting Arts*. Ventura, CA: Thor, 1972.

White, David. *Judo the Practical Way*. London: Chancerel, 1977.

KARATE

Crompton, Paul H. *Karate Training Methods*. London: Pelham Books, 1971.

Frommer, Harvey. *The Martial Arts: Judo and Karate*. New York: Atheneum, 1978.

Tegner, Bruce. *Karate and Judo Exercises. Physical Conditioning for the Oriental Sport Fighting Arts*. Ventura, CA: Thor, 1972.

LACROSSE

Boyd, Margaret. *Lacrosse: Playing and Coaching*. London: Yoseloff, 1978.

Lacrosse. Boston: Charles River Books, 1978. Wakefield, Yorkshire: E. P., 1976.

NETBALL

Netball. Boston: Charles River Books, 1978. Wakefield, Yorkshire: E.P., 1978.

Wheeler, Joyce. *Better Netball*. London: Kaye and Ward, 1970.

RACQUETBALL

Allsen, Philip, and Witbeck, Alan. C. *Racquetball, Paddelball*. Dubuque, Iowa: William C. Brown, 1977.

Reznick, John W. *Championship Racquetball by the Experts*. New York: Leisure Press, 1976.

RIDING

Churchill, Peter. *Riding from A to Z*. Poole, Dorset: Blandford Press, 1975.

Froud, Bill. *Better Riding*. London: Kaye and Ward, 1978.

Podhajsky, Alois. *Complete Training of Horse and Rider*. Hollywood, CA: Wilshire, 1977.

Stecken, Fritz. *Training the Horse and Rider*. New York: Arco, 1976.

ROWING

Burnell, Richard. *The Complete Sculler*. Marlow: Simpson, 1975.

Chant, Christopher. *Rowing for Everyone*. Newton Abbot, Devon: David and Charles, 1977.

Howard, Ronnie. *Knowing Rowing: An Illustrated Introduction to Rowing and Sculling*. London: Allen and Unwin, 1977.

Langfield, John. *Better Rowing*. New York: International Publishing Service, 1974. London: Kaye and Ward, 1974.

RUGBY

Fitness Training for Rugby. London: Rugby Football Union, 1978.

Greenwood, Jim. *Total Rugby*. London: Lepus Books, 1978.

Williams, Ray. *Skilful Rugby*. London: Souvenir Press, 1976.

SAILING

Elvstrom, Paul. *Expert Dinghy and Keelboat Racing*. New York: Time Books, 1970.

Fisher, Bob ed. *Crewing Racing Dinghies and Keelboats*. New York: Dodd, 1976.

Pinaud, Y. L. *Sailing from Start to Finish*. St. Albans, Herts, England: Adlard Coles, 1975.

SKATING

Arnold, Richard. *Better Ice Skating*. New York: Soccer, 1976.

Deleeuw, Dianne, and Lehrman, Stan. *Figure Skating*. New York: Atheneum, 1978.

Hugin, Cato, and Gerschwiler, Jack. *Technique of Skating*. London: Cassell, 1977.

SKATING—ROLLER

Arnold, Richard. *Better Roller Skating*. New York: Sterling, 1977.

Ice and Roller Skating. Wakefield, Yorkshire: E.P., 1976.

SKATING—ROLLER—contd

Shevelson, Joseph F. *Roller Skating*. New York: Harvey, 1978.

SKATEBOARDING

Brill, Allen, and Torbet, Laura. *The Complete Book of Skateboarding*. Scranton, PA: Funk and Wagnalls, 1976.

Davidson, Ben. *The Skateboard Book*. London: Sphere, 1976.

Pick, Christopher. *Safe Skateboarding*. London: Evans Bros, 1978.

Weir, La Vada. *Skateboards and Skateboarding*. New York: Simon and Schuster, 1978.

SKIING

Bennett, Maynt. *Cross-Country Skiing for the Fun of It*. New York: Dodd, 1975.

Barnett, Steve. *Cross-Country, Downhill and Other Nordic Mountain Skiing Techniques*. Seattle: Pacific Search, 1978.

Foss, Merle, and Garrick, James G. *Ski Conditioning*. New York: Wiley, 1978.

Ski Fit, Pre-Ski Exercises. London: The Ski Club of Great Britain, 1978.

The Sunday Times. We Learned to Ski. New York: St. Martins, 1976. London: Collins, 1976.

SOCCER

Owen, Brian, and Clarke, Nigel. *Beginner's Guide to Soccer Training and Coaching*. London: Pelham Books, 1973.

Ponsonby, David, and Darden, Ellington. *Soccer Fitness*. Winter Park, FLA: Anna Publications Inc., 1978.

Shepherdson, Harold, and Muckle, David S. *Football Fitness and Injuries*. London: Pelham Books, 1976.

SQUASH

Hawkey, R. B. *Improving Your Squash*. London: Faber and Faber, 1972.

Millman, A. E. *The Better Way to Play Squash*. London: New English Library, 1976.

SURFING

Klein, H. Arthur. *Surf-Riding*. New York: Lippincott, 1972.

Nentl, Jerolyn. *Surfing*. Mankato, MN: Crestwood Press, 1978.

SWIMMING

Armbruster, David A. *Swimming and Diving*. New York: Mosley, 1973.

Eady, Roger. *Modern Swimming and Training Techniques for Coach and Competitor*. London: Barker, 1972.

Hogg, John M. *Land Conditioning for Competitive Swimming*. Wakefield, Yorkshire: E. P., 1972.

Learmouth, John. *Swimming for Fitness and Fun*. Newton Abbot, Devon: David and Charles, 1976.

Wilson, Charlie. *Swimming: Learning, Training, Competing*. London: Chancerel, 1977.

TABLE TENNIS

Bloss, Margaret, and Harrison, J. Rufford. *Table Tennis*. Dubuque, IA: William C. Brown, 1976.

Leach, J. *Better Table Tennis*. London: Kaye and Ward, 1978.

Sklorz, Martin. *Table Tennis*. Wakefield, Yorkshire: E.P., 1977.

TENNIS

Gonzalez, Pancho, and Bairstow, Jeffrey. *Tennis Begins at Forty*. New York: Dial, 1978.

Haynes, Connie, et al. *Speed, Strength and Stamina Conditioning for Tennis*. New York: Doubleday, 1975.

Jones, C. M. *Match-Winning Tennis: Tactics, Temperament and Training*. New York: Transatlantic Publications, 1971. London: Faber and Faber, 1971.

Kraft, Steven. *Tennis Drills for Self-Improvement*. New York: Doubleday, 1978.

TRACK AND FIELD

Costanza, Betty. *Women's Track and Field*. New York: Hawthorn Books, 1978.

Fundamentals of Athletic Training. New York: American Medical Association, 1978.

Harper, Peter R. *Mobility Exercises*. London: British Amateur Athletic Board, 1978.

Paish, Wilf. *Introduction to Athletics*. London: Faber and Faber, 1974; New York: Transatlantic Publications, 1974.

Pickering, R. J. *Strength Training for Athletics*. London: British Amateur Athletic Board, 1975.

Shephard, Roy J. *The Fit Athlete*. Oxford: Oxford University Press, 1978.

Todd, Dr. Terry, and Hoover, Dick. *Fitness for Athletes*. Chicago: Contemporary Books, 1978

Whitehead, Nick. *Track Athletes*. Boston: Charles River Books, 1976; Wakefield, Yorkshire: E.P., 1976.

UNDERWATER SWIMMING— SNORKEL AND SCUBA

Brown, Terry, and Hunter, Rob. *The Concise Book of Snorkelling*. New York: Vanguard, 1978.

Dodds, Horace E. *Snorkelling and Skin-Diving: An Introduction*. Oxford: Oxford University Press, 1976.

Reseck, John Jr. *Scuba Safe and Simple*. Englewood Cliffs, NJ: Prentice-Hall, 1976.

Sport Diving: The Complete Manual for Skin and Scuba Divers. London/New York: Macmillan, 1978.

Underwater Swimming. Wakefield, Yorkshire: E.P., 1976.

VOLLEYBALL

Betucci, Robert ed. *Championship Volleyball by the Experts*. New York: Leisure Press, 1978.

Nicholls, Keith. *Modern Volleyball for Teacher, Coach and Player*. London: Lepus Books, 1978.

Pankhurst, Roy. *Better Volleyball*. London: A. C. Black, 1978.

WATER POLO

Juba, Kelvin. *All About Water Polo*. London: Pelham Books, 1972.

Mestre, Neville De. *Water Polo Techniques and Tactics*. London: R. Angus, 1974.

WEIGHT LIFTING

Popplewell, George. *Modern Weight Lifting and Power Lifting*. London: Faber and Faber, 1978.

Weight Lifting. Boston: Charles River Books, 1975. Wakefield, Yorkshire: E.P., 1975.

WINDSURFING

Brockhaus, Pater, and Stanciu, Ulrich. *Sailboarding*. London: Mayflower Books, 1978.

Marks, Uwe, and Winkler, Reinhart. *Windsurfing*. New York: McKay, 1976. Lymington, Hants: Nautical Publishing Co,. 1976.

WRESTLING

Carson, Ray F. *Championship Wrestling*. Cranbury, NJ: A. S. Barnes, 1974; London: Yoseloff, 1978.

Keith, Art. *Complete Book of Wrestling Drills and Conditioning Techniques*. Englewood Cliffs, NJ: Prentice-Hall, 1976.

Maertz, Richard C. *The Techniques of Championship Wrestling*. London: Yoseloff, 1978; Cranbury, NJ: A. S. Barnes, 1976.

Spackman, Robert R, Jr. *Conditioning for Wrestling*. Springfield, ILL: C. C. Thomas, 1970.